Communication Skills
for Adult Nurses

Communication Skills
for Adult Nurses

Edited by
Sarah Kraszewski
Abayomi McEwen

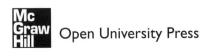 Open University Press

Open University Press
McGraw-Hill Education
McGraw-Hill House
Shoppenhangers Road
Maidenhead
Berkshire
England
SL6 2QL

email: enquiries@openup.co.uk
world wide web: www.openup.co.uk

and Two Penn Plaza, New York, NY 10121-2289, USA

First published 2010

A catalogue record of this book is available from the British Library

ISBN-13: 978-0-33-523748-7 (pb) 978-0-33-523747-0 (hb)
ISBN-10: 0-33-523748-7 (pb) 0-33-523747-9 (hb)

Library of Congress Cataloging-in-Publication Data
CIP data has been applied for

Typeset by Aptara Inc., India
Printed in the UK by Bell and Bain Limited, Glasgow

Fictitious names of companies, products, people, characters and/or data that
may be used herein (in case studies or in examples) are not intended to
represent any real individual, company, product or event.

Mixed Sources
Product group from well-managed
forests and other controlled sources
www.fsc.org Cert no. TT-COC-002769
© 1996 Forest Stewardship Council

FSC

The **McGraw·Hill** Companies

Contents

The editors and contributors

The editors

Sarah Kraszewski has worked in a variety of adult nursing roles in the NHS and higher education sector, including gynaecology, general practice nursing and sexual health. Her current role is programme leader for primary care at Anglia Ruskin University. Her professional interests are broad, but particularly focus upon primary care, women's health, non-medical prescribing and the use of communication technology in facilitating patient care. She is a registered nurse tutor, an independent and supplementary nurse prescriber and an instructing nurse in a contraception and sexual health service. Her publications have included articles and book chapters focusing on primary care and sexual health issues.

Abayomi McEwen spent 25 years as a full-time GP and is now the GP appraisal lead for West Essex Primary Care Trust. She is a part-time associate Dean for GP Postgraduate Education (Essex) and communication skills facilitator in the East of England Multiprofessional Deanery. She is involved in the training of teachers of medical communication skills as well as supporting clinicians who have been identified as needing communication skills development. She is a recognized clinical teacher at the University of Cambridge, a member of the Essex Appraisal Steering Committee, is treasurer and member of the National Association of Primary Care Educators (NAPCE) appraisal group, and was an associate lecturer at Anglia Ruskin University until 2008.

The contributors

Bernard Anderson has a professional background in adult nursing and is a registered nurse tutor. He has been working in health education since 1987, first at the Institute of Health Studies in Colchester and since 1994 as a senior lecturer at Anglia Ruskin University. He has wide professional interests including medical ethics and public health, and lectures in these to both undergraduate and postgraduate students.

Jayne Crow is a senior lecturer at Anglia Ruskin University and teaches both health and social work students on a wide range of pre- and post-qualifying courses from foundation degree to postgraduate awards. Jayne came to higher education from a career in adult nursing and has a specific interest in interprofessional learning, collaborative working and action research. Jayne's enthusiasm for the application of health psychology, particularly with regard to communication, health beliefs and concordance, has informed much of her teaching and writing. Since the mid-2000s she has been proactive in designing, delivering and researching education programmes to enhance dignity and respect in healthcare and has published and presented her work both nationally and internationally.

Graham Harris is a registered nurse and a registered nurse tutor. He has worked in a variety of roles in the NHS and the higher education sector, including as a charge nurse in an acute elderly care ward, a clinical teacher for an older people's unit and more recently as a senior lecturer at a health faculty. Currently he is working as a community nurse for Suffolk Primary Care Trust. Graham's professional interests are broad, but principally surround the care of older people, men's health and the protection of vulnerable adults. He has undertaken research into mentorship for pre-registration nursing students and more recently into nurses' perceptions of their role in the prevention and management of cases of elder abuse. He has contributed to the development of a variety of educational programmes, led the adult branch programme of an undergraduate nursing degree and participated actively in the delivery of numerous professional courses, study days and workshops. His publications include papers related to men's health and end of life care. He is currently awaiting the publication of a chapter within a nursing textbook on health promotion in later life.

Jackie Jones was a practice nurse for over 20 years and as a result has had a long interest in nurses' development and educational needs. Since the early 2000s she has become involved in practice nurse education, working as a trainer teaching the asthma diploma and as a nurse representative on the PCG board. From there Jackie moved into primary care education full time and also became involved in the East of England Deanery working as an associate director for nursing as part of the multiprofessional team. She was successful in introducing into Essex the Practice Nurse Apprenticeship Scheme and the Preceptorship and Assessment Tool for Practice Nurses. She contributed to the Working in Partnership Programme (WiPP) for practice nurses and healthcare assistants, and has more recently been working as a professional adviser for primary care nurses at the East of England Strategic Health Authority.

Vivian Jellis is currently working as a community matron for Peterborough Primary Care Trust. Her previous roles have included working as a case manager, a consultant nurse, a senior lecturer in primary and community care and as a midwife. Her current role requires the use of advanced clinical assessment skills and communication skills, coordinating and liaising with health and social care colleagues. Her current interests include team working within an integrated health and social care provider unit and communication within and between teams.

Mary Northrop is currently a senior lecturer at Anglia Ruskin University teaching social policy and sociology for nursing and healthcare professionals. She has been involved with teaching both pre- and post-registration nurses and in developing and delivering pre-professional courses. Mary completed a masters in medical sociology at Royal Holloway College and prior to that a combined degree in sociology and literature at Kingston University. She has worked as a nurse in both adult and mental health settings and is a registered nurse tutor. Her professional interests include the sociology of risk, public health, and the development of new roles in the NHS. Her publications include contributing to a book chapter on amplification of risk and a chapter for a mental health text book on physical healthcare.

Paula Sobiechowska started her career in higher education in 1998 and has worked with health and social care students at all stages of their educational journey, from pre-qualifying courses through to post-qualifying graduate programmes. She has interests in work-based learning, reflective learning (particularly that which arises out of expressive or creative media) and, increasingly, the learning experience of overseas/international students. Her current role is as director of learning and teaching at Anglia Ruskin University.

Jill Toocaram is currently the programme leader of the common foundation year for DipHE and BSc pre-registration nursing students at Anglia Ruskin University. Jill is qualified as an RNMH (RNLD), an RGN and is a registered nurse tutor. She has over 30 years experience, including working on a female adolescent unit and in the community, and has been an active member of the RCN Learning Disability Forum. After completing two part-time degrees and spending many years facilitating students in practice, Jill moved into the education sector full time and is in the privileged position of being able to influence and develop the nursing curriculum to help make sure no group is marginalized or forgotten in a time of constant change and cultural diversity.

Foreword

We are often accused within the health profession of acting with paternalism, and the fight for information, the experience and processes of healthcare organizations can cause additional stress and anxiety for patients on top of any health problems they may have.

Healthcare in the modern NHS is challenging and demanding, and as health professionals we are required to provide a high quality of service to our patients. They expect and deserve the best we can offer, and key to that service is the ability to communicate effectively and with compassion.

My years as a nurse have taught me that communication is a topic that is often disregarded but remains fundamental to the quality of care we deliver. The difference we can make in people's lives is often measured by how we communicate and interact with them, making their experience of healthcare a positive one, rather than the number of technological interventions prescribed. This reminds me of a time many years ago, as a student nurse. I was required to care for a very ill patient during one long dark night, so I spent as much time as was possible with them on that first night after a major surgical procedure. My role was to monitor all the technical equipment but in the course of the night I spent a great deal of time holding the patient's hand and reassuring them. Over the following days and weeks the patient insisted on telling everyone that I had been the source of their recovery. Now I knew that wasn't the reality, but the patient obviously felt that the level of communication we had shared that night had somehow contributed to their sense of wellbeing. The words of Rudyard Kipling, in a speech made to the Royal College of Surgeons in 1923, sum up what the patient meant: 'Words are, of course the most powerful drug used by mankind.'

However, it is not only the words we use but the way we deliver them that is also important, to ensure that the people we are dealing with understand what is being said. As health professionals we are in a privileged position to care for those who are at their most vulnerable. It is vital that we listen carefully to what they have to say, so that we can support and care for them.

This book will prove invaluable to students and mentors alike as it sets out clearly the essence of communication. Each chapter deals with a particular aspect of communication within the health service and there are plenty of examples and prompts which allow the reader to reflect on their own practice. It is also designed as an aid for teaching, with useful discussion prompts provided at key junctures. By communicating effectively we are able to make a difference to people's lives, which I believe is an essential part of being a health professional.

Jackie Jones

Preface

Nursing is known as the 'caring profession', and nurses spend their working days communicating with patients and other healthcare professionals. It has been recognized that communication is the fundamental skill that underpins every human interaction, and nurses, like all other healthcare professionals, need to learn effective communication skills to ensure they can communicate appropriately with service users and other healthcare professionals. Successful delivery of healthcare relies upon both conscious and unconscious communication skills and these are an essential component of the pre-registration nurse training curriculum. The daily encounters of the qualified nurse require effective communication as a core skill and this is recognized by the Nursing and Midwifery Council (NMC) as one of the essential skills clusters in nurse education. These skills can be taught, must be learnt, and can be improved upon throughout a nurse's career.

There are many good communication skills textbooks available. This book is intended to be a practical everyday guide to communication skills for nurses and other health professionals working with adult patients. It aims to be a text that will support both student nurses learning their craft and a suitable reference for qualified nurses undertaking continuing professional development (CPD), or acting as mentors to student nurses.

The chapters have been written by a range of health professionals, each looking at communication from a different perspective, providing a rich, layered and multifaceted approach to core communication skills, supported by many years of experience. Examples of both good and poor practice are included to provoke reflection and facilitate integration of theory and practice. The vignettes and patient perspectives are fictitious, but have been created from the real-life experiences of the authors, to ensure the book relates to everyday practice, and provides a practical hands-on approach to improving patient care. There is of course an overlap between chapters, as each communication encounter will draw in a range of issues, but this also serves to underpin the importance of these skills.

We have included an introduction to consultation skills because evolving nursing roles increasingly require the development of such skills post-registration. Other chapters cover issues such as dignity and respect, assessment, conflict resolution, traversing barriers, team working and the influence of information technology (IT) on our daily working practice. Each chapter can be read independently, but we have included links to other chapters to ease navigation where a particular aspect of communication is being studied. A book of this size cannot cover all aspects in depth, but we hope it provides a useful introduction to the core skills and will encourage readers to reflect on their practice.

Every health professional will, at one time or another, be on the receiving end of healthcare services. What will be remembered? The faultless adherence to guidelines? Or being treated politely, kindly and with dignity and respect? Patient surveys recurrently show that people wish to be listened to and included in the decision-making about their care. We hope that this book will help you to consider the patient's experience and strive to give all patients a positive experience of healthcare.

Sarah Kraszewski and Abayomi McEwen

Acknowledgements

For help with producing this text we would like to thank Dave Kraszewski for his time, patience, IT skills and critical eye throughout. We would also like to thank the authors of the individual chapters who have worked selflessly to meet the deadlines and responded to our feedback gracefully.

We are grateful to Drs Jonathan Silverman and Julie Draper for permission to reproduce the Calgary Cambridge Framework and to use their material on breaking bad news.

We would like to thank RNID for permission to reproduce information from their website, www.rnid.co.uk. RNID works to create a world where deafness or hearing loss do not limit or determine opportunity, and where people value their hearing. It raises awareness of deafness and hearing loss, promotes hearing health, provides services and engages in social, medical and technical research.

RNID Information Line
Telephone 0808 808 0123 (freephone)
Textphone 0808 808 9000 (freephone)
Fax 020 7296 8199
19–23 Featherstone Street
London EC1Y 8SL
informationline@rnid.org.uk
www.rnid.org.uk

We are grateful to the Social Care Institute for Excellence (www.scie.org.uk) for permission to reproduce an adaptation of the Payne and Scott Supervision Model (1982).

Communication: fundamental skills

Abayomi McEwen and Graham Harris

Clinical competence is the ability to integrate several important clinical skills – history-taking, problem-solving, assessment and knowledge – all underpinned by effective communication. Communication with others is an innate skill that is variably developed in all human beings. This chapter introduces students to the exploration of the communication that occurs between health professionals and patients. It aims to provide students with a basic understanding of different modes of communicating and to enable critical analysis of health professional–patient interactions. Students will also be introduced to the concept of a structure for interactions and consultations, with activities and topics for reflection to assist the concepts discussed. The skills learned from this chapter are transferable to many areas of work including communication in teams, teaching and social interaction.

Learning outcomes

By the end of this chapter you should be able to:
1. Describe the attributes of effective communication.
2. Develop a structured approach to patient encounters.
3. Develop the skills to critically analyse interactions with patients, whether observed or undertaken by the student.

Introduction

Communication is often taken for granted as it is a part of daily life. In the health-care setting particularly, it can have disastrous outcomes when it is ineffective. It is accepted that history-taking is far more important than examination in making a diagnosis (Hampton *et al.* 1975), yet it is only recently that communication has been recognized as a clinical skill that, like all other clinical skills, should be formally taught (Duffy 1998).

Terminology: assessment or consultation?

Given that effective communication has long been recognized as the cornerstone of high-quality care, it follows that patient assessment – the first part of the nursing process – requires practitioners to be skilled communicators (McCabe and Timmins 2006; Field and Smith 2008; Kydd 2009). This is particularly important when initiating a patient encounter. At these times, anxiety and uncertainty are often high – even among people experienced in using the healthcare system. Sensitive, responsive and thoughtful communication helps to address the anxieties and ensure that the care the patient subsequently receives meets both their needs and aspirations.

What is assessment?

The term 'assessment' is used so frequently in healthcare that it is easy to assume everyone understands it in the same way – an assumption far from the truth. Some, for example, see assessment as a very formal and structured activity involving interviewing and examining a patient, identifying signs and symptoms, proposing a diagnosis and possibly treatment or a treatment plan. Others see it as a less formal but ongoing process whereby data about a patient is gathered and analysed as the patient–practitioner relationship develops. Different models may be adopted and these influence not only the type of information collected, but *how* it is collected.

Some would argue that every nurse–patient encounter involves assessment. In fact, even a simple 'hello' can be assessed. Just one word can reveal a vast amount about the person who has spoken it, from their mood or need to engage others, to their understanding of time and whether it is an appropriate moment to speak. We hear a voice and a message, not just words but emotions, accents and tones. Sometimes we can even guess at the thoughts behind them! This type of assessment tends to go on subconsciously, but should not be underestimated since it involves the subtle, almost intuitive reading of cues – the essence of effective communication (Benner 1994; RCN 2004; Fairly and Closs 2006).

Generally, the term 'assessment' is used in nursing to describe the first phase of the nursing process, where data is collected so a plan of care can be developed and goals set (Miller 2002; Uys and Habermann 2005). Clear examples of this include initial assessments on hospital admission, or a first encounter with a community nurse. However, nursing assessment is not a 'once-only' procedure, it is a dynamic, continuous and developmental process.

The widening scope of practice means that nurses are increasingly involved in more complex interactions with patients (Lloyd and Craig 2007). Practice nurses, nurse practitioners in various specialties and community nurses are examples of nurses whose interactions with patients could be described as 'consultations'. Thus, as in clinical practice, assessment and consultation are used interchangeably in this chapter and the activity below will help to illustrate the point.

Activity

Identify members of the interprofessional team within your current placement. For example, speech and language therapist, physiotherapist, doctor, nurse practitioner.

- Ask each one what they call the interaction they have with patients.
- Ask if they could summarize the elements of the interaction and what they think is different to what you would do as a student or newly-qualified nurse.
- Write down their answers and reflect on the similarities and differences.

Modes of communication

Communication is usually divided into two categories, verbal and non-verbal. There is also an equally important third category, known as 'paralinguistic' or 'para-verbal'. All three modes of communication are usually used together. Mehrabian's (1981) research into body language and non-verbal communication found that only 7 per cent of a message is conveyed by the actual words we speak, 38 per cent by paralinguistic features (e.g. tone and pitch) and 55 per cent by other non-verbal factors.

Verbal communication

In this category of communication, the actual words used are considered. Nurses need to choose their words carefully so that they match the patient's ability to understand them. This is particularly important when giving information to patients. It is very easy to slip into medical jargon, especially when explaining a complex situation which may only be partially understood by the general population. The possibility for misunderstanding is increased when either party does not have English as a first language, and is even more likely when neither speak English fluently. Even when English is spoken fluently, accents, dialects, euphemisms, colloquialisms and acronyms (see Chapter 3) can obscure the understanding to the point where the patient may be disappointed, alienated or, worse still, their healthcare may be compromised (Lloyd and Craig 2007).

Patient perspective
A 65-year-old widow has just started a new relationship and had sexual intercourse for the first time after many years which resulted in vaginal bleeding. As she waits to see the practice nurse in the walk-in centre, she may be thinking: 'How am I going to tell the young nurse what's wrong with me and how it happened? I hope she doesn't say she can't deal with it and that I have to see the doctor . . .'

Activity

When the widow sees the nurse she says, 'It's me down belows.'

- What do you think the patient means?
- Can you think of any other colloquialisms or euphemisms that could obscure something that you would need to tell the patient? Write them down and check with a colleague from another part of the UK what they understand by these terms.

Paraverbal communication

Paraverbal communication can be described as the attributes that 'dress' the words. For example, the volume at which an assessment is conducted might have to be high because the patient is hard of hearing. However, it is possible that the nurse may raise their voice in response to a patient speaking loudly, which could inflame an already tense situation. The volume of the consultation is important as it is already difficult in many healthcare settings to achieve privacy.

The tone of voice is also important as this can impart an unintentional message which reflects how the sender is feeling, despite trying to be neutral. For example, when a long-standing patient says to the nurse, 'You must be so fed up seeing me!', the nurse may try to answer politely but the tone of voice may convey boredom. The emphasis on a particular word could have significant meaning. Reflect on the conversation below and think about what meanings there might be to the patient's response.

Reflection point

Consider what you might be able to infer from the following.

Nurse: I'm wondering if your father has ever hurt you?
Patient: No, not *him*!

Speed of speech is another characteristic that can emphasize the meaning provided by the words. For example, it is quite normal for adolescents to speak very quickly and use jargon to the point where adults find it difficult to understand them. In a different context, for example on a mental health ward, fast speech is described as 'pressured speech'.

Health professionals often do not tolerate pauses and silences when interacting with patients. This may be due to time pressure, but it is still vital to recognize the need to develop sufficient rapport for a 'companionable silence'. Silences often seem longer than they actually are, yet it is important to appreciate that health professionals ask complex questions which patients need time to reflect on.

Non-verbal communication

The terminology used in describing non-verbal communication is not rigid and there will be overlap between the descriptions given here and those in other chapters. Non-verbal communication can be described as those messages that are transmitted without using any words. Non-verbal communication is very powerful – a look, a gesture, facial expression or touch can set the tone for an encounter before a word is uttered. Many researchers agree that the receiver of the message will usually pay more attention to the non-verbal than the verbal communication. Thus as health professionals it is essential to consider the non-verbal messages we transmit, and to be sensitive to those we receive from others.

Positioning is another issue that is not always sufficiently considered. Health professionals are now advised to arrange the assessment area so that they are the same height as patients in order to minimize perceptions of superiority or inferiority. In hospital settings, staff often stand by the bedside while they discuss sensitive issues with a patient. While time is often short, it is worth making the effort to find a chair and sit down next to the patient, at least for important discussions such as care and treatment options. Ambulatory patients have more control and may position their seat closer than the health professional finds comfortable. They may use it to be threatening or familiar, depending on how they perceive they will get what they want. Chapter 7 addresses communication skills that will help in such challenging situations. However, it is important for individuals to consider safety issues when designing consultation areas. Many consulting rooms are arranged so that the patient is between the health professional and the door. On the other hand, if there are several chairs in the room the patient may choose a seat at a distance from the consulter. While this may be a simple mistake, it should alert the health professional to pay more attention to the patient's feelings about personal space.

Gestures may convey nervousness or mean very little unless read as part of the whole communication. McNeill (2005) showed that gesturing is an active part of both speaking and thinking. Gestures may be culturally influenced, thus it is worth spending time to interpret them correctly as they may reveal what a patient is thinking but not necessarily saying.

Reflection point

Have you observed different cultural behaviours? For example:

- Men kissing each other on the cheek in greeting.
- People expecting to shake hands.
- Being asked by relatives not to tell a patient when the diagnosis is terminal.

Can you think of any others?

Much has been written about eye contact, but care must be taken not to put meaning where it does not exist. In western culture it is acceptable, indeed expected, that eye contact will be made. In some cultures it is rude for younger people to make eye contact with their elders, while in others men and women do not make eye contact unless they are very close relatives. Generalizations are dangerous and it is perfectly reasonable for a western woman to not make eye contact because she is shy, not because she is depressed.

'Body language' includes all the attributes described above as part of non-verbal language. It is also used to describe the message given by the way the body is used when communicating. Thus, in addition to the behaviours described above, whether the legs are crossed or not, whether the head is nodded or shaken, can give messages to the other person.

Touch is another form of non-verbal communication that needs to be used judiciously. Appropriately expressed, it can convey empathy more eloquently than words. However, healthcare professionals are increasingly wary of touching patients when it is not part of recognized treatments such as bathing, applying dressings and giving an injection, in case it is misconstrued. There is a dearth of research evidence on which to base touch as a therapeutic communication (Gleeson and Timmins 2005). Thus student nurses will have to rely on their instincts and develop experience to judge when it is prudent to touch patients as an expression of empathy.

Active listening

Active listening is a core skill in communicating with patients. It is important to contemplate what the patient's words and body language really say, and to *listen* to the answer. The simple wisdom of the old adage, 'when communicating, never forget we have two ears, two eyes and only one mouth' remains as sound as ever. To develop trust and gather meaningful information generally involves giving full attention, asking open-ended questions, listening carefully and concentrating on what is being said. A useful mnemonic for this is SOLER –see Table 1.1.

Listening skills need to be developed so that patients can tell their story in sufficient detail to facilitate good quality care. Often described as *active listening*, the

Table 1.1 Becoming a better listener

There are many ways to communicate to a person that we are giving them our full attention. These simple behaviours can help us to create the comfortable, secure and relaxed atmosphere that enables a patient to talk freely.

The acronym SOLER is used to summarize some of the important behaviours – as follows:

- **S = squarely** face the person. Facing them in this way makes your posture say 'I am ready to listen to you'.
- **O = open** your posture. This is a non-defensive position – it shows you are open to the other person's words. Crossed arms and legs can represent less involvement.
- **L = lean** forward to the other person. This again shows that you are listening.
- **E = eye contact** maintained. As you listen, use your eyes to show you are looking at the person. In this way, they know you are concentrating on what they are saying.
- **R = relax** while attending. It is entirely possible to be both concentrating and relaxed. In turn, this will help the other person to feel comfortable and relaxed.

nurse is not required to sit silently while the patient rambles for an indefinite period of time. The listener needs to give non-verbal messages which encourage the patient to share, while feeling safe and cared for. The patient also needs to know that the listener will not judge and will be honest. While listening, the information received needs to be processed, sorted and used to plan the next step of the interaction while demonstrating that the patient has the listener's full attention. Interestingly, 'silent' and 'listen' are anagrams of each other, and this corroborates Morton Kesley's statement that listening is being silent in an active way (Kelsey 1976).

In summary, it is important for the nurse to appreciate that communication consists of sending messages between the patient and the healthcare professional. There could be many factors in both parties that result in the message that is received being very different from the intended message sent. It is by learning to read the non-verbal language of patients, and the health professional being aware of the non-verbal messages they might be transmitting, that truly effective communication can occur.

Consulting effectively with patients

The consultation is the unit of work undertaken by any healthcare professional, whether it is very task-focused or involving complex diagnostic and prescribing skills. It has been calculated that a healthcare professional, working full-time for most of their professional life, could undertake approximately 150,000–200,000 consultations with patients. While each interaction is different, healthcare professionals have found that there are some common occurrences in each interaction. This thinking has led to the idea that if an overarching structure for a generic interaction could be developed, it would be a useful tool to discuss, analyse and improve all exchanges. These structures are known as models, frameworks or maps.

Using a model or framework for patient assessment

In order to achieve an effective assessment, most nurses use a framework, model or written prompt to guide them. Of course, very experienced nurses may assess a patient without immediate reference to any document or guidelines, but even so, aspects of a nursing model are likely to be used, albeit implicitly.

The frameworks used take many forms but their role is to clarify thinking so that each patient can be assessed in a systematic and comprehensive way. Most hospitals or organizations have pre-printed assessment documentation that reflects a model and provides such a framework (Kozier *et al.* 2008).

One commonly used framework derives from the Roper, Logan and Tierney (2000) model, and requires nurses to assess each patient in relation to 12 activities of living (ALs); in fact, the model contains five 'conceptual' components altogether, and all of these are illustrated in Table 1.2.

According to Roper *et al.* (2000), this model promotes individualized, systematic nursing. However, there are many other models and it is worth investigating them. For example, Orem's (1991) and Roy's (1976) models are both relevant to adult nursing, offering different perspectives and insights for practice.

Table 1.2 Components of the Roper, Logan, Tierney model for nursing

1	Activities of living (ALs)	Maintaining a safe environment Communicating Breathing Eating and drinking Eliminating Personal cleansing and dressing Controlling body temperature Mobilizing Working and playing Expressing sexuality Sleeping Dying
2	A lifespan continuum	People may require nursing at any point of the lifespan – from birth to death
3	A dependence/ independence continuum	We need to assess the patient's level of dependence in each AL so that goals can be set to help towards independence or acceptance of dependence
4	Factors influencing the ALs	Each AL should be considered from five perspectives – biological, psychological, sociocultural, environmental and politico-economic
5	Individuality in living	Each individual is unique and nursing must take account of this when assessing and planning care.

Interestingly, not everyone sees nursing models as useful and there has been some contention over their value. Some argue that models tend to be 'reductionist' in nature, encouraging nurses to adopt a 'checklist approach' to assessment (Kelly 1988; Kenny 1993; van Maanen 1990).

One criticism levelled at the Roper, Logan, Tierney model is that it concentrates on *physical* aspects of patient care (Ellson 2008). However, the issue is one of interpretation; while the ALs may seem physiologically based, if the model is used as designed, then broader psychosocial perspectives are addressed.

Activity

Select two of the ALs from the Roper, Logan, Tierney model.

- For each, identify how you might assess a patient, including observations you would make and questions you would ask.
- Make a list of your ideas.
- Now consider the five perspectives: biological, psychological, sociocultural, environmental and politico-economic.
- Look at your list and see how you addressed each of these perspectives. What changes might you make as a result?

Having a framework may well be essential to guide thinking and the type of information gathered, but the question remains: how should assessment be conducted?

Other models

There are several other consultation models (e.g. see www.commscascade.medschl. cam.ac.uk) and it is useful to get to know one or two of them in depth. Using these models at the beginning of a career will enable health professionals to develop a personal style based on good practice and underpinned by evidence.

There are broad similarities between models, and the Calgary Cambridge Framework (Silverman *et al.* 2005) is one that can be applied to most healthcare professions. The Calgary Cambridge Framework is used mainly by doctors (70 per cent of the 33 medical schools in the UK now use it). However, it has also been discussed and introduced into nursing and pharmacy schools. The basic framework of this model is shown in Figure 1.1, but the Appendix on page 20 of this chapter contains further information which provides more detail (reproduced with the kind permission of the authors). The full model goes on to list all the evidence-based skills and explains their practical application. While the model at first sight looks

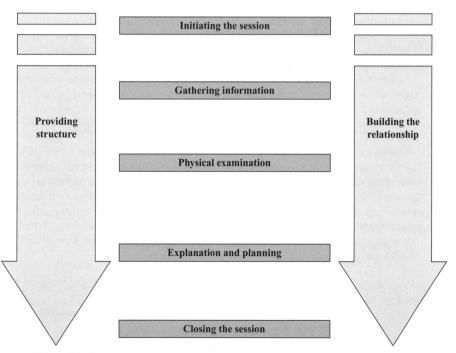

Figure 1.1 The enhanced Calgary Cambridge guide to the medical interview – the basic framework

complicated, it is very detailed and extensively referenced. It is comprehensive and therefore useful throughout a clinical career.

It is not possible in this book to do more than highlight the most important skills that will provide the student with a firm foundation. *Skills for Communicating with Patients* (Silverman *et al.* 2005) gives further details about individual communication skills. The subsequent chapters of this book will help the student build on this basic introduction. The above frameworks will now be used as the basis for exploring specific skills for effective communication in assessing/consulting with patients. The two main activities that run throughout a consultation are explored first.

Building relationships

It can be daunting for patients to see health professionals arrive with a clipboard and set of notes. Not knowing what to expect or being concerned that others will overhear can inhibit communication, so it is important to explain briefly that assessment involves discussion of personal information that will be kept confidential.

A comfortable environment is essential – preferably a private and soundproof room (Barnes 2009). The nurse should position themselves at the patient's level, so there can be good eye contact and the 'safe' closeness that is necessary to share personal information. Sharing is an important concept here – the emphasis is on establishing a rapport where patients feel they are collaborating with the nurse, not being subjected to an interview or test. Although many patients expect nurses to take the lead, 'supported participation' and partnership usually make for the most effective care, so it is often worth showing patients the relevant forms, and in some cases sitting side by side to address the various requirements.

General questions about name, address and other biographical details are always essential, so they are the usual starting point. Within seconds, however, a conversation can begin – asking a person how they like to be addressed, for example, will demonstrate respect for their choices and can pave the way for a relaxed conversation.

The more experienced nurses become, the less they need to refer to pre-printed forms. In fact, as confidence develops, nurses can listen and observe more, concentrating less on documentation and much more on what the patient says and how they appear or are behaving. This does not mean that documentation is not a vital part of assessment – quite the reverse. Record-keeping is critical to effective communication (Ellson 2008). However, if nurses spend time actively listening, observing the patient and conversing with them, then the records produced are likely to be a more accurate reflection of the patient's needs.

Vignette	Shared understanding?
	Nurse: Hello Mr Peters. My name is Nurse Smith, I'm going to do a holistic assessment and find out your nursing needs. Is that okay? [Nurse looks down at paper, pen poised]

Patient:	All right Nurse Smith. I see ... nursing needs ... I see ... a 'whole' assessment?
Nurse:	Yes. First of all – can you tell me about your environment?
Patient:	My environment? You mean our house? Where we live?
Nurse:	Yes, your house. I mean, do you have stairs? And is your toilet upstairs? That sort of thing.
Patient:	Well it's a house but we have moved downstairs now. We have a bathroom downstairs. My wife has arthritis, you see, and ... it's much easier.
Nurse:	I see. So is it just you and your wife?
Patient:	Yes. It's just us two ...
Nurse:	Do you need help?
Patient:	Help? Help at home? With the house and all that? Well, our daughter does our shopping. We manage, you know. We get by. Our neighbour does the lawn.
Nurse:	Yes, yes, I see. Okay. [Nurse looks down, writes on sheet, then looks up] Do you have any carers?
Patient:	No, like I said, our daughter does all the heavy shopping. My wife doesn't really want anyone else. Our daughter is good, you know. She calls in nearly every day.
Nurse:	Okay. So I will write 'daughter looks after your care needs at home'.
Patient:	Well, she does help out but I still manage for myself really.
Nurse:	Good. How about your breathing? Do you have any problems?
Patient:	My breathing? Sorry? Say it again, nurse ...
Nurse:	Any shortness of breath? [Nurse looks at chart at bottom of the bed, writes on notes]
Patient:	No. Not really. Nothing much really.

Activity

This activity would be most effective undertaken as a trio. One nurse to role-play the patient, one to play Nurse Smith and a third as an observer. Use the transcript above to conduct the initial role play. After the role play, the 'patient' should feed back on how it felt, then the nurse and finally the observer. Swap roles and try different ways of playing the nurse to see how it alters the patient's behaviour and the way the nurse feels. Specifically, what is the effect of ignoring or picking up cues?

From the transcript above, it is easy to see how several poorly phrased questions 'aimed at' a patient can ultimately become a series of missed opportunities and provide almost meaningless details. The key, therefore, is always to listen *actively* to the patient.

Effective questioning is a skill worth developing and the use of both open and closed questions is useful in the assessment process. An *open question* will enable the patient to start where they like and that may provide very useful information. An open question will enable a patient to offer their own perspectives, opinions and feelings, which will support the healthcare professional in undertaking assessment. *Closed questions* are also useful and can be used to elicit particular details or explore specific issues. They would generally follow the use of open questions in an assessment process.

Reflection point

'Would you mind telling me about your pain?' is an example of an *open question*. 'How long have you had your pain?' is an example of a *closed question*. Think about the different answers you would get to each type of question and how they might affect your relationship with a patient you have just met.

Picking up cues

Attending to the comfort of the patient, picking up on non-verbal cues and managing your own non-verbal cues all contribute to the building of rapport. Patients may, for example, give non-verbal cues that they are very uncomfortable discussing sensitive matters on an open ward, so the veracity and depth of information obtained may be poor. Physical discomfort such as being too short to sit comfortably in the chair provided may not be easily resolved, but acknowledging that there is a problem coupled with an apology that it cannot be rectified will make the person feel valued. This links with preserving the dignity of the patient, discussed in Chapter 3.

The choice of words and phrasing is important. Using expressions like 'holistic assessment' can be disconcerting, and ambiguous questions should be avoided. It is usually better to use the patient's own words, keeping language simple and concise. How much clearer to say, 'Please tell me about where you live?' and 'I am asking some questions to get to know you and see how we can help.'

Looking at the transcript above once again, Nurse Smith could have found out much more by following the cues that were given. For instance, by following up on the point about the daughter, she could have asked whether she lives nearby or if she has her own family. Mr Peters may then have felt that the nurse was genuinely interested, and would have been more likely to disclose more. It would have certainly showed that the nurse was listening – hearing what the patient wanted to say, not just what had to be asked.

Of course, assessment does not only involve questioning and interviewing. Sometimes we need to examine the patient and this needs to be explained so that the patient can give consent. For example, if the patient has a wound or requires blood pressure measurement, these observations are part of the assessment process (Kozier *et al.* 2008).

Health professionals are often rushed, tired and hungry. They may be irritated because they feel that they are working harder than other colleagues or have issues that may be detrimental to their performance. Unless a nurse is aware of these feelings and the impact they may have on the patient, the patient may react negatively without the nurse understanding why. In his five-step consultation model, Roger Neighbour (2005) urges the health professional to stop momentarily and ask if they are in good enough shape to move to the next patient. Issues left over from a previous consultation or encounter may be a block to building rapport in the current one.

Providing structure

When undertaking consultation and assessment, using a structure to guide the process can also help the health professional develop their skills in time management. This ensures that the time a nurse has with a patient is used effectively and important elements are not overlooked. A useful skill here is called 'signposting'. It can be described as holding the patient's hands (metaphorically speaking) and leading them through the consultation step-by-step. This helps to avoid repetition and signals a move to another topic or another activity, such as being examined.

Examples of signposting

From the patient:

- 'There are three things I wish to discuss with you today, nurse ... '
- 'When you've finished changing my dressing, there's something I'd like to ask you.'

From the nurse:

- 'We need to finish our discussion soon so that the blood I have taken will catch the next collection.'
- 'If you're happy that I have answered all your questions about your cough, we can move on to talk about you going home.'

The Calgary Cambridge Framework describes five steps of the consultation which, supported by building rapport and providing structure, help the nurse to develop a holistic approach to patients. The important skills in each of these stages are now briefly highlighted.

Initiating the session

It is often said that judgement should not be made on first impressions. Nevertheless, the initial welcome a patient receives will leave a lasting impression; getting it right is important. That does not mean that people will not forgive an obviously busy nurse if, for example, they have to wait a few minutes. All the same, simple courtesies really do matter – a smile, being shown to a seat, a 'Hello, how are you?'

spoken with genuine concern all convey a respect that only helps in developing relationships (see also Chapter 3).

Furthermore, these courtesies should never be dismissed as 'the basics'. Repeatedly, ombudsman reports highlight inadequate communication as a major source of complaints about healthcare, and invariably communication failures are at the root of things when treatment goes wrong (Oxtoby 2005; Health Service Ombudsman 2008).

There may be many reasons for this, but in terms of assessments and admissions it is important to acknowledge how overwhelming the experience may be for a patient. Aside from the often complex problems patients may be experiencing, today's healthcare environments are increasingly busy and pressurized. Some are full of sophisticated pieces of technology that bleep, alarm and distort perceptions of what is happening. In such a dehumanizing environment, people may feel bewildered and isolated. At the risk of stating the obvious, staff who smile, introduce themselves and engage patients with appropriate eye contact and an open posture are likely to make a real difference as far as patients are concerned.

Vignette   A home visit
Consider the following situation.

Mr Carter has arrived at the doctor's surgery and needs to find out how he can request a home visit for his wife, as he has been unable to get through to the surgery by telephone. When he arrives, two receptionists are sitting at the reception desk. One receptionist is talking on the telephone and the other is looking intently at her computer screen. The practice nurse is also in reception but has her back turned, filing a set of notes. As Mr Carter approaches the desk, the receptionist on the telephone holds up her hand in a 'stop' gesture and then points to the touch-screen where patients are expected to 'check in' on arrival for their appointments. She continues her telephone conversation but nudges the other receptionist to get her attention – unsuccessfully. Mr Carter waits a couple of minutes before the other receptionist sees him and asks how she can help him.

Patient perspective
Mr Carter might be thinking, 'I really can't cope with this. My Anne is really unwell and I need to get back to her. Now I am here they don't even want to speak with me. I don't need to use the machine as I don't have an appointment. I bet they'll tell me the doctor is too busy to come home to Anne. I think I'll hang around in the corridor and see if I can catch the nurse for a quick word.'

Reflection point
Think about how patients and visitors are greeted in the service in which you work.

Setting the agenda

Having greeted a patient, the next part of assessment involves establishing any immediate or 'emergency' needs. These obviously take precedence, although much depends on the issues bringing the patient to the care service. A person with severe pain or shortness of breath, for example, will clearly be unable to answer lots of questions and in some circumstances it may be inappropriate to do much more than a visual assessment and baseline observations before treatment is commenced.

For the majority of patients, however, it is entirely appropriate to begin a more in depth assessment shortly after or as part of the initial meeting. With introductions made, the next step may need to be the negotiation of an agenda as it is important to work out and agree what can reasonably be covered in the time available. The patient needs to be involved in agreeing what is going to be dealt with, otherwise the health professional will experience that sinking feeling in the pit of their stomach as the patient says, 'While I'm here nurse ...'. Often the health professional will work on the first problem presented by the patient. Starfield *et al.* (1981) found that in 50 per cent of visits patient and doctor do not agree on the main presenting problem. Their findings confirm that practitioner–patient agreement about problems is associated with a better outcome as perceived by the patient. In addition, they indicate that practitioners also report better outcomes under the same circumstances.

Sometimes the patient may separate symptoms and present them individually, while together, as a clinical pattern, they may suggest a single diagnosis. For example, eliciting a list of symptoms such as tiredness, nausea, slight right upper abdominal pain, dark urine and light-coloured stools immediately leads one to think of liver-related disorders. Delving deeply into the first symptom of tiredness at the outset could mean that the health professional does not get all the other symptoms in good time and the consultation travels down a very different path.

Gathering information

Once the agenda is set, it is important to explore each item in turn to develop and test the patient's thoughts about a provisional diagnosis. Most health professionals are good at learning the specific 'scientific' questions that relate to a symptom. These 'systematic questions', as they are called, are very useful as they give clinicians a structure that helps them practise safely and not miss any dangerous symptoms. However, it is also really important to understand how the patient views what is going on. Disease as diagnosed is very different from illness as lived, and people respond differently. The acronym ICE (ideas, concerns and expectations) is often used glibly without putting the skills required into practice.

Activity
With a colleague, ask each other the following questions and discuss the effect on each of you and what you think the effect might be on your patients.

- 'What are your ideas, concerns and expectations?'

- 'It would help me to understand the problem better if I knew what you are thinking about all this?'
- 'Is there anything concerning you about what is going on?'
- 'Is there anything in your mind that you think we might do to help this problem?'

Finally, it is important to put all the information gleaned into the patient's context, so that the treatment suggested is accepted by the patient. For example, telling a man to take time off work without realizing he is the sole breadwinner, with an employer who does not pay sick leave, just will not work. It is vital to learn enough about the patient as a person by gathering appropriate background information. If the information required is very personal, it helps to tell the patient why and to signpost and perhaps normalize that part of the consultation. For example, in a sexual health clinic: 'I am now going to ask you a series of personal questions that we ask everyone with your kind of problem. It will help us decide what further tests you may need, if you need any at all . . . '

Physical examination

Nurses in their daily roles examine patients. It may be an everyday activity such as inspecting a wound or taking readings of vital signs, or indeed, for those working in extended roles, listening to the patient's chest or undertaking a vaginal examination prior to taking a swab or cervical cytology. The patient needs to give explicit consent. The nurse needs to explain to the patient what the examination entails and obtain the patient's agreement. If there is a procedure linked with the examination then that needs to be explained before starting. The nurse needs to consider whether the offer of a chaperone is appropriate (NMC 2008).

Chapter 3 will help the student embed the concepts of treating patients with dignity before during and after the examination. Offering help with dressing sensitively, for example, may be overlooked when time is short. It is often assumed that an elderly person will welcome help with undressing, but if this is not the case they are robbed of their dignity. This scenario may diminish any rapport that may have been built up in the earlier part of the interaction.

Explanation and planning

This is the part of the assessment where the health professional collates the information, comes to an idea of what is going on and needs to enter into a discussion with the patient about what might be wrong, what can be done, and what the patient thinks and will agree to, so that a plan can be made. This can be the most time-consuming part of the consultation/assessment as it is what the patient is really waiting for – or fearing.

Apart from using plain language without jargon, the nurse has to ensure that the patient does not get lost and has ample opportunity to ask questions, while avoiding being patronizing.

Health professionals need to practise explaining risk until they find a form of words that patients can relate to. Many patients access the internet prior to their appointment or admission which makes this part of assessment much more of a discussion and negotiation than it used to be. When the patient and the health professional are speaking in equal proportion, or if the patient is speaking more, it means that the patient is engaged in the development of the plan and therefore it is more likely to be executed. A lecture ending with 'Any questions?' leaves the stunned patient with very little understanding or recall.

Information must be broken up into manageable chunks, with time for the patient to digest and question before moving on to the next bit. It is also necessary to find out where the patient is starting from, otherwise unnecessary information may be given, without addressing the patient's real information needs.

Activity

Mrs Brown has just been diagnosed with type 2 diabetes and has been sent to the nurse to learn how to manage her disease. Diabetes is a huge topic for a patient to learn about.

- Think for a minute about how you would undertake this task. It would be helpful to role-play with a colleague.
- Think about how you would start and how would you decide what to tell her.
- If she were obese, as is likely, it might be obvious to you that she has to lose weight. But how do you know that is her priority?

Closing the session

This section overlaps with the previous one. Having developed a plan for managing the problem with the patient, a plan for the future needs to be made. What does the patient need to do? When does the patient need to come back, if at all? 'Safety netting' is a phrase that is often bandied about, but to be performed well it has to be more detailed than, 'If it doesn't get better, come back.' Most patients are not nurses and may not realize when their symptoms become dangerous. Equally, and detrimentally for the healthcare system, if they do not have clear guidance they may come back too soon, straining resources.

Patient perspective

Alfonso Vadini, a 46-year-old man, passed blood in his urine and went to his local accident and emergency (A&E) department because he was so alarmed. His father died of prostate cancer and Alfonso knew he had blood in his urine.

He saw a nurse practitioner who diagnosed a urine infection, gave him five days' supply of antibiotics and told him to see his GP if it did not get better. Six days later, his urine was still dark, but there was no blood. On reflection Alfonso realized he had been feeling tired for a few months. He might have been thinking, 'I wish the hospital had not been busy that night, I could not say how worried I was. The nurse might have thought I was being weak. What did she mean by "better"? I am "better" but not quite well. I don't want to waste anybody's time'.

It is also very useful to offer clearly-written evidence-based information for the patient to take away. Encouraging the patient to read the information and note any questions or concerns to discuss on a return visit is not only reassuring for the patient, but also helps to build rapport. It gives the patient permission to 'not understand or remember fully'. It can also empower patients to take more control of a chronic condition if they have a written plan – for example, asthma management plans which guide the patient to increase or reduce medication according to the severity of their symptoms.

Once the interaction has ended, it is important for the health professional to take stock momentarily to see if there is anything that might be carried over into the next consultation. Is there a fear that something was forgotten or should have been done differently? Was a practical skill mastered after many failed attempts? Is a comfort break needed?

If all these aspects are not addressed, the next assessment can be a disaster, because of tensions or emotions within the health professional. While it may seem a luxury, this brief self-check could save a lot of time in the future.

Conclusion

Effective communication with patients is a huge topic, underpinned by a vast body of research. It is a skill set that needs to be continually brushed up and developed throughout any health practitioner's career. This chapter has only highlighted the most important topics and concepts for the student nurse:

- learn to listen actively;
- explore the use of a nursing model – this will give a structure for learning, working and updating;
- always try to keep the patient's perspective in mind;
- be aware of how your communication skills can be affected by your own emotions and thoughts;
- identify potential learning from every human interaction regardless of the setting.

References

Barnes, J. (2009) Health promotion in sexual health 2: nurses' role in engaging with clients, *Nursing Times*, 105: 19.

Benner, P. (1994) *From Novice to Expert – Excellence and Power in Clinical Nursing Practice*. London: Addison Wesley.

Duffy, F.D. (1998) Dialogue: the core clinical skill, *Annal of Internal Medicine*, 128: 139–41.

Ellson, R. (2008) Assessment of patients, in R. Richardson (ed.) *Clinical Skills for Student Nurses: Theory, Practice and Reflection*. Devon: Reflect Press.

Fairly, D. and Closs, S.J. (2006) Evaluation of a nurse consultant's clinical activities and the search for patient outcomes in critical care, *Journal of Clinical Nursing*, 15: 1106–14.

Field, L. and Smith, B. (2008) *Nursing Care: An Essential Guide*. Harlow: Pearson Education.

Gleeson, M. and Timmins, F. (2005) A review of the use and clinical effectiveness of touch as a nursing intervention, *Clinical Effectiveness in Nursing*, 9(1–2): 69–77.

Hampton, J.R., Harrison, M. J., Mitchell, J. R., Prichard, J. S. and Seymour, C. (1975) Relative contributions of history-taking, physical examination, and laboratory investigation to diagnosis and management of medical outpatients, *British Medical Journal*, 2(5969): 486–9.

Health Service Ombudsman (2008) Improving public service: a matter of principle, www.ombudsman.org.uk/pdfs/improving_public_services.pdf (accessed 25 May 2009).

Kelly, L. (1988) The ethic of caring: has it been discarded? *Nursing Outlook*, 36: 17.

Kelsey, M.T. (1976) *The Other Side of Silence: A Guide to Christian Meditation*. Mahwah, NJ: Paulist Press.

Kenny, T. (1993) Nursing models fail in practice, *British Journal of Nursing*, 2(2): 133–6.

Kozier, B., Erb, G., Berman, A. *et al.* (2008) *Fundamentals of Nursing: Concepts, Process and Practice*. Harlow: Pearson Education.

Kydd, A. (2009)Values: what older people told us, in A. Kydd, T. Duffy and F. Duffy (eds) *The Care and Wellbeing of Older People: A Textbook for Healthcare Students*. Devon: Reflect Press.

Lloyd, H. and Craig, S. (2007) A guide to taking a patient's history, *Nursing Standard*, 22(13): 42–8.

McCabe, C. and Timmins, F. (2006) *Communication Skills for Nursing Practice*. Basingstoke: Palgrave Macmillan.

McNeill, D. (2005) *Gesture and Thought*. Chicago: Chicago University Press.

Mehrabian, A. (1981) *Silent Messages: Implicit Communication of Emotions and Attitudes*. Belmont, CA: Wadsworth.

Miller, T.W. (2002) *Keeping Informed: Nurses Taking the Lead*. Philadelphia, PA: W.B. Saunders.

Neighbour, R. (2005) *The Inner Consultation: How to Develop an Effective and Intuitive Consultation Style*. Reading, MA: LibraPharm Ltd.

Nursing and Midwifery Council (NMC) (2008) *The Code: Standards of Conduct, Performance and Ethics for Nurses and Midwives*, www.nmc-uk.org.uk (accessed 11 March 2010).

Orem, D. (1991) *Nursing Concepts of Practice*, 3rd edn. New York: McGraw-Hill.

Oxtoby, K. (2005) Reaching a clear understanding, *Nursing Times*, 101: 20.

RCN (Royal College of Nursing) (2004) *Nursing Assessment and Older People: A Royal College of Nursing Toolkit*. London: Royal College of Nursing.

Roper, N., Logan, W.W. and Tierney, A.J. (2000) *The Roper, Logan, Tierney Model for Nursing Based on Activities of Living*. Edinburgh: Churchill-Livingstone.

Roy, C. (1976) *Introduction to Nursing: An Adaptation Model*. Upper Saddle River, NJ: Prentice Hall.

Silverman, J., Kurtz, S. and Draper, J. (2005) *Skills for Communicating with Patients*. Oxford: Radcliffe Medical Press.

Starfield, B., Wray, C., Hess, K. *et al.* (1981) The influence of patient-practitioner agreement on outcome of care, *American Journal of Public Health*, 71(2): 127–31.

Uys, L.R. and Habermann, M. (2005) The nursing process: globalization of a nursing concept – an introduction, in M. Habermann and L.R. Uys (eds) *The Nursing Process: A Global Concept*. Edinburgh: Churchill Livingstone.

Van Maanen, H. (1990) Nursing in transition: an analysis of the state of the art in relation to the conditions of practice and society's expectations, *Journal of Advanced Nursing*, 15: 914–24.

Appendix

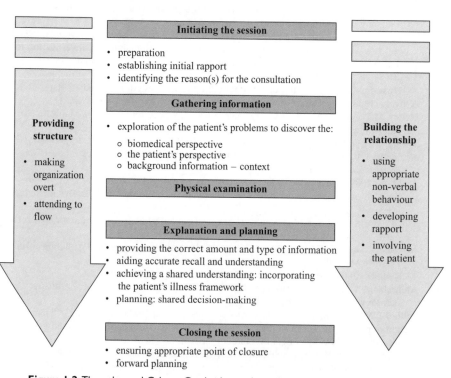

Figure 1.2 The enhanced Calgary Cambridge guide to the medical interview – the expanded framework (Silverman et al. 2005)

Gathering Information

Process skills for exploration of the patient's problems

☐ patient's narrative

☐ question style: open to closed cone

☐ attentive listening

☐ facilitative response

☐ picking up cues

☐ clarification

☐ time-framing

☐ internal summary

☐ appropriate use of language

☐ additional skills for understanding patient's

perspective

Content to be discovered

The biomedical perspective (disease)
Sequence of events
Symptom analysis
Relevant systems review
Effects on life
Feelings

Background information - context
Past medical history
Drug and allergy history
Family history

The patient's perspective (illness)
Ideas and beliefs
Concerns
Expectations

Figure 1.3 An example of the interrelationship between content and process
(Silverman et al. 2005)

Patient's problem list
Exploration of patient's problems

Medical perspective–disease	*Patient's perspective–illness*
Sequence of events	Ideas and beliefs
Symptom analysis	Concerns
Relevant systems review	Expectations
	Effects on life
	Feelings

Background information – context
Past medical history
Drug and allergy history
Family history
Personal and social history
Review of systems

Physical examination

Differential diagnosis – hypotheses
Including both disease and illness issues

Physician's plan of management
Investigations
Treatment alternatives

Explanation and planning with patient
What the patient has been told
Plan of action negotiated

Figure 1.4 Revised content guide to the medical interview (Silverman et al. 2005)

2 Communicating with adult patients: beyond the fundamentals

Graham Harris and Abayomi McEwen

In this chapter, the need for nurses (and other health professionals) to observe and *listen actively* forms a recurrent theme, underpinning the skills described in Chapter 1.

Learning outcomes

By the end of this chapter you should be able to:
1 Extend the generic skills explored in Chapter 1 to dealing with adult patients.
2 Introduce the concept of holistic care.
3 Develop strategies for handling sensitive topics with patients.
4 Develop effective strategies for communication with families and relatives.

Introduction

It is essential to develop and refine communication skills when working with adult patients in sensitive situations. The *Concise Oxford Dictionary* describes adults as being 'mature' or 'grown up'. However, it is important to be aware that becoming a patient can be a stressful experience and that not everyone will respond in an adult way. Consideration is therefore given to becoming a better observer and listener, especially in relation to patient assessment. Basic empathy and sympathy and their role in assessment are discussed along with breaking bad news, advocacy, 'sensitive' issues and the provision of comfort and reassurance.

Patient assessment: a holistic approach

Like any health assessment, nursing assessments are undertaken to identify a person's needs and problems – both actual and potential. Objective and subjective data are required, so that it is possible to understand what the patient is experiencing, how it is affecting them and the issues that are their priorities (Holland 2008). However, the focus is not only health and medical problems – we are also concerned with broader issues and often sensitive ones, in terms of how a person lives their life, their wishes and goals. Without being invasive, the aim is to address the patient's 'total' physical, psychological and social wellbeing – to achieve a *holistic assessment*.

Holism is an important philosophy in healthcare and its use in nursing has been widely promoted (Silva and Rothbart 1984; Serkis and Skoner 1987; Rousseau and Saillant 1988; Milligan and Stevens 2009). The word itself derives from the Greek '*holos*' which means 'whole' – but it also relates to healing which, in turn, derives from the word '*kailo*' – meaning 'whole' or 'intact' (Ayto 1990).

According to Smuts (1926), our understanding of human beings should be based on the fundamental assumption that all individuals 'as whole beings' are *different from* and *more than* the sum of their parts (Pearson *et al.* 2005). To translate this into nursing practice, holism means that we seek to understand patients as more than just people with medical conditions or illnesses – we aim to appreciate them as unique individuals with social and psychological needs as well as physical ones. Hence, effective communication when undertaking assessments requires skills in complex relationship-building and information-gathering.

Empathy and sympathy

Empathy is an important communication skill. It is particularly helpful in building a relationship (Breckenridge and Blows 2008) when dealing with sensitive issues. The terms 'empathy' and 'sympathy' are frequently used interchangeably in healthcare, but there is a significant difference in meaning which is straightforward to describe but can be awkward to implement: sympathy involves feeling *for* a person, whereas empathy involves feeling *with* them (Egan 1975, 2002).

To put this into context, when a person is sympathetic, they may feel sorry about another person or a problem the person is experiencing. However, when they show empathy (as shown in the patient perspective below), they consider how they would feel if they were in the person's position – a far more helpful activity since it can be used to help the other person explore and express their feelings too.

Patient perspective

> *Nurse:*   I can see that the changes you are going to have to make in your life to manage your diabetes are going to be really difficult for you.
>
> *Patient:*   It's not the dieting and increased exercise that concern me, I'm worried about going blind like my aunt did.

This contrasts significantly with a sympathetic response which would only offer commiseration, not an opportunity to bring feelings out into the open and discuss them. In patient assessment, empathy is necessary because it allows the nurse to understand the patient's perspective and to get a feeling for their world (Egan 2002; McCabe and Timmins 2006). From such a standpoint, it is much easier to address the real issues and offer support. Building empathic responses into assessments and other aspects of nursing is only achieved through practice.

Activity

Consider the following examples and ask yourself:

- What you might say if you were being sympathetic.
- How you would demonstrate empathy.

Case 1

Your best friend has just returned from a job interview at which they were unsuccessful. The job they applied for meant a lot, not just a higher salary but the chance of promotion in a few years' time. Your friend seems close to tears.

Case 2

A patient has been waiting for over an hour to see a member of medical staff who has been called to an emergency. You have to reschedule their appointment. As you approach, you notice the patient's arms are folded, and they seem very angry.

Dealing with sensitive issues

Assessment and communication in nursing inevitably involve dealing with personal information, sometimes discussing issues that are sensitive in nature. Hence, nurses must show respect, use tact and diplomacy, and take care around the boundaries people use to protect themselves. First and foremost, self-awareness on the nurse's part is essential. The ability to establish trust combined with finely-tuned listening and observation skills is critical (Harris 2007). To make this less abstract, consider the vignette below.

Vignette   Family matters

Robert Thurston, a self-employed painter and decorator, has been admitted today with a diagnosis of acute chest infection. He is aged 64, married to Margaret, who is 20 years his junior and has an 18-year-old son called Peter from a previous marriage. Mr Thurston is an ex-smoker, weighs 100 kilograms and is 1.72 metres tall.

He was diagnosed with asthma five years ago and has had two related admissions. For the past few days he has had difficulty managing his self-care because of the chest infection. His respiratory rate is now around 24 per minute and he appears comfortable while sitting upright in bed. He has a productive cough and has requested the commode twice since his arrival.

Mrs Thurston has spoken with staff and says they are both worried about the financial implications of Robert being off work. The couple recently moved and were hoping to retire soon, handing over the business to Peter. Peter, however, has stated that he intends to go to university before following into the business. Just as she is about to leave the ward, Mrs Thurston also says that she thinks her husband needs a laxative.

Activity
- Having read through the above, identify the questions you would like to ask Mr Thurston.
- Make use of the activities of living listed in Chapter 1, Table 1.2, to group your questions into a list.
- From your list, identify the issues that would be the most sensitive.
- Ask yourself if there are any questions that you would not wish to ask and, if so, why that might be the case.

A sensitive issue can be defined as any matter a person finds difficult to discuss publicly or causes them some degree of embarrassment or emotional discomfort. However, knowing *which* issues are sensitive to a person is not always straighforward. Different people find different issues sensitive – almost any personal topic has the *potential* to be 'sensitive'. In fact, few people feel comfortable discussing private areas of their lives, even with their partners, closest friends and family.

Patient perspective
A patient like Mr Thurston might be thinking, 'I hate being in hospital. I am sure my coughing keeps the others awake. The stuff I cough up is nasty and it's really embarrassing for me to have to spit it into a pot. I feel for the nurses having to look at it . . . I just wish I was well enough to go home and do things for myself . . .'

Working in healthcare and regularly meeting people with health problems, it is easy to become desensitized to these issues. However, we must never forget the personal nature of the matters we discuss and how this can threaten dignity if not handled with care.

Some areas are, of course, known to be sensitive. Cultural mores dictate the acceptable or unacceptable areas for public discussion. For example, we tend not to talk about using the toilet, personal sexual activity or even personal hygiene. In nursing, because these areas may be associated with health, we may have licence to mention them – but only when there is clear relevance to health problems and nursing care (Field and Smith 2008; Kozier *et al.* 2008) (see Chapter 1).

Looking at the activities of living, areas such as 'expressing sexuality', 'eliminating' and 'dying' may immediately stand out, but all the others are potentially sensitive too. Take for example the activity of personal cleansing and dressing. A discussion of this may impart values about frequency of washing or changing of clothes. Questions about cleaning teeth or washing hair can be similarly awkward, especially if the patient wears a wig or dentures and feels concerned about their appearance.

Careful observation and listening will usually give a cue that a topic is difficult territory for the patient. There may be, for example, a change in the person's body language, their posture may close or seem guarded, they may avoid eye contact or blush. Other obvious signs include inappropriate laughter, uncomfortable coughs or deliberate changes of subject.

Awareness of our own boundaries is important too. Knowing what we feel happy to discuss sometimes helps us to understand the information others are happy to share. The framing of questions is crucial – if people are asked open-ended questions and are not rushed, they may respond more freely. Using a non-judgemental approach coupled with active listening is important.

Knowing how to tackle embarrassment is also important. Sometimes a very matter-of-fact approach is helpful. This means being direct but respectful – never badgering or labouring a point when someone is obviously embarrassed.

Sometimes, a topic should be left until a person has had a chance to compose themselves or think through their answer. It is quite acceptable to say something like, 'I noticed you needed the commode twice today and wondered if you have a problem with your bowels?'. If the patient says a hurried and uncomfortable 'No', accept this (it is something you can return to later), thank them and say something along the lines of, 'Okay, but please let us know if you need any help.'

In many ways, effective communication in sensitive areas is about giving people permission to say something they believe is impolite or indelicate, or may show them in an unfavourable light. That does *not* mean health professionals should tolerate lewd or offensive language, it simply means respecting the individual's dignity, taking their problems seriously and responding with maturity and genuine concern.

Another of the issues raised in the scenario was the Thurstons' concerns about financial matters. The reason this may be sensitive is that Mr Thurston's wife raised the issue, not him. It may be that he is neither concerned nor embarrassed to discuss this. The problem, however, is one of collusion. Mrs Thurston is asking staff to be aware of a possible problem, but it is not clear if her husband has agreed to this.

The tensions arising from this type of scenario are all too common in healthcare. On the one hand, relatives and carers are great sources of information and contribute significantly to the assessment process (Holland 2008; Duffy 2009). Respecting their input is essential – nurses need to show that they value it and listen carefully to any concerns they raise. However, on the other hand, nurses should avoid situations where patient information is discussed away from the patient or without the patient's consent. There is a fine line between giving comfort to a relative and breaking the trust a patient has shown in the professional responsible for their care.

Sometimes nurses can feel out of their depth when dealing with sensitive issues. It is therefore important to know how and when to refer an issue to others with more expertise. Nurses are in a privileged position; patients often share intimate information, sometimes without any prompting. However, if the issues raised require a level of expertise beyond our own, we must use others within the team – either more experienced nurses or colleagues from other professions.

One final point in this section – there is a need to carefully think through the information asked *of* patients. They are under no obligation to tell staff more than they wish, and although we may be involved with very personal matters, this does not give us the right to pry. Assessment may cover areas from dying to expressing sexuality, but this does not mean that we can blunder in and question indiscriminately.

Breaking bad news

Bad news is distressing for both the receiver and giver. Health professionals need to be aware that there may be huge difference between their idea of bad news and the patient's. The patient's attitude to 'news' will be coloured by their health beliefs and it is important to find out early the impact of the news given. For example, one patient receiving a diagnosis of prostate cancer may be devastated because several members of their family have died of the same complaint, but another may not be as concerned as the health professional, because his experience is that two of his friends had treatment and are still alive. However, to give bad news requires a level of self-control that is comforting to the receiver; it is about being calm but not cold, restrained but not unfeeling, gentle but direct, sensitive but honest.

It is recognized that breaking bad news is not a task to be assigned to just any team member. It requires skilled, even expert, communication techniques (DHSSPSNI 2003). Nevertheless, all staff working when patients or families are given unpleasant news may become involved in some way or at some point. Furthermore, staff do not develop expertise in these situations by being excluded from them. Supported involvement of junior staff is necessary so they have the opportunity to develop their skills.

Firstly, we need to be clear what is meant by 'bad news'. Sometimes people think this just relates to terminal disease or dying. However, the issue is more complex – bad news can relate to many different types of suffering and losses, and may include any of the following:

- a diagnosis of a terminal disease, for example, widespread cancer;
- the death of a loved one – including pets and friends;

- the loss of a limb or loss of function within a limb/organ/loss of a sense (e.g. sight, hearing);
- confirmation of a chronic disease, for example Parkinson's disease.

According to the DHSSPSNI (2003: 3), the key feature of bad news is that it is a message that has 'the potential to shatter hopes and dreams leading to very different lifestyles and futures'. Of course, the issue is not which type of loss is more or less worthy of support – all are worthy. The issue is to deliver the news in a compassionate way – not giving false hope but not conveying hopelessness.

Before giving bad news, staff need to consider numerous issues, from how well they know the patient and how much the patient knows about the situation, to where and when the news will be broken and who will provide aftercare and support (see Table 2.1).

Table 2.1 Breaking bad news

Preparation
- allow enough time; ensure no interruptions
- use a comfortable, familiar environment
- invite spouse, relative, friend, as appropriate
- put aside own 'baggage' and personal feelings wherever possible

Beginning/setting the scene
- summarize where things have got to date, check with the patient
- calibrate how the patient is thinking/feeling

Sharing the information
- assess the patient's understanding first: what the patient already knows, is thinking or has been told
- gauge how much the patient wishes to know
- give warning first that difficult information is coming. For example, 'I'm afraid it looks more serious than hoped'
- give basic information, simply and honestly; repeat important points
- do not give too much information too early; don't pussyfoot but do not overwhelm
- give information in small chunks
- watch the pace, check repeatedly for understanding and feelings as you proceed
- use language carefully – giving regard to the patient's intelligence, reactions, emotions: avoid jargon

Being sensitive to the patient
- read the non-verbal cues; face/body language, silences, tears
- allow for 'shut down' (when patient turns off and stops listening) and then give time and space: allow possible denial
- keep pausing to give patient opportunity to ask questions
- gauge patient's need for further information as you go and give more information as requested. In other words, listen to the patient's wishes as patients vary greatly in their needs

(continued)

Table 2.1 Breaking bad news (*continued*)

- encourage expression of feelings, give early permission for them to be expressed: 'how does that news leave you feeling?', 'I'm sorry that was difficult for you', 'you seem upset by that'
- respond to patient's feelings and predicament with acceptance, empathy and concern
- check understanding of information given - 'would you like to run through what you are going to tell your family?'
- be aware of unshared meanings
- do not be afraid to show emotion or distress

Planning and support
- identify a plan for what is to happen next
- give hope tempered with realism ('preparing for the worst and hoping for the best')
- ally yourself with the patient ('we can work on this together'); partnership with the patient/advocate of the patient

Follow-up and closure
- summarize and check with patient
- don't rush the patient to any decisions
- identify support systems; involve relatives and friends
- offer to see/talk with spouse or others
- make written materials available
- ongoing support after the news has been broken

(Adapted from Skillscascade 2002)

The communication skills needed when breaking bad news are varied, but in particular they involve active listening and picking up on the cues of body language, speaking in a clear and concise way, avoiding jargon and clichés and, finally, offering empathy, warmth and respect.

Communicating with people for whom English is not their first language

As nurses we may often come into contact with patients who speak little or no English. Hence, we need to be aware of how we can communicate in these situations while still providing good quality care, support and comfort that crosses any language barriers.

The first response, when there has been no time for a planned approach, involves using non-verbal communication techniques like smiles, gestures and other body language. Much can be communicated in this way and it may even be appropriate to consider simple drawings to try to explain actions. If the patient speaks a small amount of English or the nurse speaks a little of the patient's language it may be possible to form simple sentences, but time should be taken over this. The patient should be faced, so good eye contact can be maintained, and background noise should be minimized to allow for clarity.

For more complex communication, other resources are needed. As Field and Smith (2008) note, most organizations have contact with trained interpreters and a list of emergency translators. A 'language line', where a translator communicates with both nurse and patient over the telephone is also usually available.

If a translator is used and they are present, staff must remember that it is the patient, not the interpreter, with whom they are communicating. Hence, when asking questions and listening to responses, eye contact should be maintained with the patient. The nurse should speak to the patient, not the translator. As always, body language and non-verbal cues are critical to success. The aim is to put the patient at their ease (not just the translator) (see Chapter 6). It is important to clarify the role of an interpreter. Some may be trained advocates as well. Both the patient and the healthcare professional need to know the exact role and capabilities of the person supporting the patient, whether they are a professional or a relative.

Vignette   Breaking bad news

Monique is a 22-year-old French woman who has been staying with Angela, her English pen-pal. Sadly, the friends have been involved in a serious accident and have both sustained multiple injuries. Angela has been admitted to the intensive care unit as she is unconscious and it is likely that she will require amputation of one of her legs. Monique has been admitted to the orthopaedic ward as she has fractured a femur. Although her physical condition has been stabilized, Monique is obviously distressed and, despite understanding basic English, she calls out and mostly responds in French. She knows that her friend is in the intensive care unit but is unaware of the extent of Angela's injuries. Some of the nursing staff speak a little French but the interpreter has contacted the ward to say she cannot get to the hospital for another hour. Monique's family have been informed of her accident and Angela's parents are expected shortly.

Activity

Make a list of the communication issues that you think are involved in the case of Monique and Angela.

Clearly, the scenario concerning Monique and Angela involves complex communication issues, not only related to language barriers but also to breaking bad news. In the circumstances it would be appropriate for a member of staff who speaks some French to remain with Monique until she is calmer and her condition less critical. The presence of a nurse in such situations is essential. The nurse may need to adopt the role of advocate and will certainly need a range of skills including empathy and the ability to give reassurance while continuing assessment and delivering the care Monique needs.

At some point, the precise nature of Angela's injuries will have to be communicated to Monique. However, the nursing staff will not only have to consider Monique here – the families and friends of both girls will need very skilled and sensitive communication as well.

Advocacy

Advocacy is another important concept in this context. Definitions usually describe it as 'speaking up for' or defending the rights of another (Kozier *et al.* 2008). In healthcare, the need for advocacy is often quite marked. Illness, frailty, fear, a lack of confidence or information can render a patient vulnerable and, moreover, unable to speak with the confidence or articulacy that many situations require (Henderson 2009).

These situations are not necessarily life-threatening or dramatic; on the contrary, they often involve everyday issues. Nevertheless, it is important not to underestimate them. Helping someone who cannot understand a menu to choose their meal is sometimes as important as helping them to understand their medication or treatment. As adults we all have the right to make choices and decisions; as nurses we sometimes need to defend those rights for our patients. We must ensure they are not ignored or overlooked.

In the case of Monique, her language skills mean she may have difficulty asserting her rights. The nurse acting as her advocate should therefore try to provide her with the information she needs in order to be able to make informed decisions.

Table 2.2 Advocacy skills

- *Listening skills* – taking time to listen in a confidential and safe environment
- *Empathy* – showing genuine interest in the person's point of view; being non-judgemental and open-minded
- *Knowing the system* – understanding people's rights and entitlements, having knowledge of local services and procedures
- *Negotiation skills* – being assertive without being aggressive, having sound communication skills across a range of audiences
- *Tenacity* – being persistent, trying all available options
- *Independence* – being free from conflicts of interest – not being swayed from support of the person by other people or agencies

(Adapted from Henderson 2009)

has spoken with them about the proposed amputation. Angela's father appears stunned – he is sitting at the bedside holding his daughter's hand. Angela's mother is distraught; she is crying and waving her arms about in a state of shock. A nurse has been asked to give support to Angela's parents.

- What do you think the nurse could do to provide comfort?

Providing comfort and reassurance

Giving comfort is a key nursing function and there are many different interpersonal and communication skills involved. While the spoken word can be very supportive, it is mostly the tone of speech that is soothing. Reassurance may therefore be less about what the nurse says and more about the way they say it. A soft or gentle voice, not demanding immediate decisions or in-depth answers, can be very comforting. Using the person's name or chosen form of address is important here too – it shows respect – letting the person know that they are the focus of attention.

Possibly more important, however, are non-verbal communication skills, such as active listening and the ability to recognize increasing tension and anxiety in others. An unhurried nurse with an open posture who shows genuine concern in her facial expression is obviously more likely to appear approachable and comforting to someone who is troubled than a busy nurse who seems tired and stressed herself.

Touch is another aspect of non-verbal communication that has a role in reassurance. Touch via a supportive hand on a shoulder or forearm may convey acceptance, warmth and caring (Chang 2001). Sometimes the slightest touch can trigger an outpouring of emotion, and this may be of great benefit. It must be acknowledged, however, that not all people like being touched, so caution must be exercised. Usually it is possible to see by a person's body language if this is the case (see Chapter 1).

Sometimes, the presence of a nurse is enough to help a distressed person. Comfort, in such instances, comes from knowing there is another person to share their feelings with – someone they trust. Actions such as accompanying a patient to another department or perhaps just sitting next to them in companionable silence are very much appreciated.

In fact, knowing when to speak and when to be silent is a critical skill. Sometimes silence says more than words. Accepting and feeling comfortable with it may take experience, but it is important not to 'jump in to fill the gaps' when a person is trying to think something through or just needs time to be quiet.

If the patient is distressed, it may be tempting to try to find quick, easy solutions in an attempt to resolve their issues. Yet, wherever possible, the person should be encouraged to find their own solutions. The best communicators facilitate the patient's own decision-making and problem-solving. Sadly, this may sometimes mean helping them to accept that there is not always an immediate solution.

Heron (1989) has devised a useful system for categorizing different types of interpersonal interventions that can be applied to the processes of giving comfort and support. This system is outlined in Table 2.3.

Table 2.3 Heron's six categories of intervention

AUTHORITATIVE INTERVENTIONS

1 *Prescriptive* – interventions that involve giving advice and direction
2 *Informative* – interventions about providing information
3 *Confronting* – interventions that challenge or raise the patient's awareness of their own behaviours or attitudes

FACILITATIVE INTERVENTIONS

4 *Cathartic* – interventions that encourage the expression of emotions
5 *Catalytic* – interventions that encourage the patient to explore their own behaviours and thinking and 'draw out' insights
6 *Supportive* – interventions that seek to validate and affirm the worth of the patient and their qualities/actions

A final point: the most important thing nurses bring to work each day is themselves. Being your 'natural self' or the 'real you' is the key to effective communication. Rewarding relationships will nearly always be the result – a fine achievement for all concerned.

Conclusion

Nurses today work in an environment of ever more complex technology, rapid-pace treatments and increasing patient expectations. The need to possess and make use of a wide range of communication skills has never been greater. The skills discussed in this chapter are some of the most important ones to meet that need. From patient assessment to the provision of comfort and reassurance, consistent messages are evolving and include:

- listening actively;
- observing carefully;
- generally speaking less than the patient;
- using empathy rather than sympathy to build relationships so that patients feel safe to discuss sensitive issues;
- understanding that patients' relatives need care, reassurance and empathy;
- developing advocacy skills – a necessary component of a nurse's communication skill set.

References

Ayto, J. (1990) *Dictionary of Word Origins*. St Ives: Columbia Marketing.

Breckenridge, S. and Blows, W. (2008) Communication between patients, carers and healthcare professionals, in J. Spouse, M. Cook and C. Cox (eds) *Common Foundation Studies in Nursing*, 4th edn. Edinburgh, Elsevier.

Chang, S.O. (2001) The conceptual structure of physical touch in caring, *Journal of Advanced Nursing*, 33(6): 820–7.

DHSSPSNI (Department of Health, Social Services and Public Safety, Northern Ireland) (2003) *Breaking Bad News: Regional Guidelines*. Belfast: Department of Health, Social Services and Public Safety.

Duffy, F.J.R. (2009) Involving relatives and carers, in A. Kydd, T. Duffy and F. Duffy (eds) *The Care and Wellbeing of Older People: A Textbook for Healthcare Students*. Devon: Reflect Press.

Egan, G. (1975) *The Skilled Helper*. California: Brookes/Cole.

Egan, G. (2002) *Exercise in Helping Skills: A Manual to Accompany the Skilled Helper*, 7th edn. London: Brookes/Cole.

Field, L. and Smith, B. (2008) *Nursing Care: An Essential Guide*. Harlow: Pearson Education.

Harris, G. (2007) Male sexual dysfunction, in T. Bishop (ed.) *Advanced Practice Nurse*. Edinburgh: Elsevier.

Henderson, R. (2009) Older people and advocacy, in A. Kydd, T. Duffy and F. Duffy (eds) *The Care and Wellbeing of Older People: A Textbook for Healthcare Students*. Devon: Reflect Press.

Heron, J. (1989) *Six-Category Intervention Analysis*, 3rd edn. Guildford: University of Surrey Human Potential Resource Group.

Holland, K. (2008) An introduction to the Roper–Logan–Tierney model for nursing, based on activities of living, in K. Holland, J. Jenkins, J. Soloman and S. Whittam (eds) *Applying the Roper–Logan–Tierney Model in Practice*, 2nd edn. Edinburgh: Elsevier.

Kozier, B., Erb, G., Berman, A. *et al*. (2008) *Fundamentals of Nursing: Concepts, Process and Practice*. Harlow: Pearson Education.

McCabe, C. and Timmins, F. (2006) *Communication Skills for Nursing Practice*. Basingstoke: Palgrave Macmillan.

Milligan, S. and Stevens, E. (2009) Palliative care, death and bereavement, in A. Kydd, T. Duffy and F. Duffy (eds) *The Care and Wellbeing of Older People: A Textbook for Healthcare Students*. Devon: Reflect Press.

Pearson, A., Vaughan, B. and Fitzgerald, M. (2005) *Nursing Models for Practice*. Oxford: Butterworth Heinemann.

Rousseau, N. and Saillant, F. (1988) Alternative therapies in nursing: more than a fashion, in R.A. Johnson (ed.) *Recent Advances in Nursing*. Edinburgh: Churchill Livingstone.

Serkis, J. and Skoner, M. (1987) An analysis of the concept of holism in nursing literature, *Holistic Nursing Practice*, November/December: 61–9.

Silva, M. and Rothbart D. (1984) An analysis of changing trends in philosophies of science on nursing theory, *Development and Testing Advances in Nursing Science*, 6(2): 1–13.

Skillscascade (2002) A framework for breaking bad news, www.skillscascade.com/badnews. htm (accessed 25 May 2008).

Smuts, J.C. (1926) *Holism and Evolution*. New York: Macmillan.

3 Communication: the essence of care

Jayne Crow

This chapter considers how nurses communicate the dignity and respect that is the essence of healthcare and is the right of all service users in healthcare settings. Through the use of vignettes and examples it will encourage reflection on the attitudes, behaviour and situational influences that may compromise effective communication of these values, and will seek to focus the reader's attention on strategies to enhance this key aspect of care.

Learning outcomes

By the end of this chapter you should be able to:
1 Describe the interpersonal skills used in healthcare settings to convey dignity and respect to others.
2 Identify and reflect on the attitudes and situational factors that underpin treating people with dignity and respect in a healthcare setting.
3 Identify strategies for enhancing the dignity and respect afforded to people in a healthcare setting.

Introduction

What exactly are we trying to communicate in a healthcare setting? This will depend on the context in which we are working and our role within it. Perhaps it involves giving information, breaking news, asking or answering questions, making an agreement, trying to reassure, calm or motivate. The list is endless and each activity demands particular skills and strategies from practitioners. However, there is one underlying requirement for all communication engaged in by healthcare professionals: we must convey that we value the patient or carer as an individual person who deserves to be treated with dignity and respect. This must be achievable even in the most difficult and trying circumstances. It is what makes a professional health carer and is 'the essence of care'.

Patient perspective
'As you walk in the door of the hospital your dignity goes out of the window.'

Communicating dignity and respect in healthcare

The need to raise the profile of dignity and respect in healthcare has been increasingly recognized by government in recent years. A key milestone came with the publication of *The Essence of Care: Patient-focused Benchmarking for Health Care Practitioners* (DH 2003).

This policy and guidance aims to embed good person-centred practice into the care of NHS patients and is organized around ten groups of benchmarks. The two groups of particular relevance to this chapter are the 'Benchmarks for communication between patients, carers and healthcare personnel' and the 'Benchmarks for privacy and dignity'. The agreed outcomes of these two groups are shown in Table 3.1

Table 3.1 The agreed outcomes for the communication, privacy and dignity benchmarks (DH 2003)

The patient-focused outcome for the communication benchmarks is that:
    Patients and carers experience effective communication, sensitive to their individual
      needs and preferences, that promotes high quality care for the patient.
The patient-focused outcome for the privacy and dignity benchmarks is that:
    Patients benefit from care that is focused upon respect for the individual.

The Essence of Care document, available online at www.dh.gov.uk, also contains best practice factors against which you can measure practice in your own area and these may be useful to promote discussion with your colleagues in order to raise standards of care. You could record your reflections on these discussions and put them in your portfolio of placement experience or continuing professional development (CPD).

What do we mean when we talk about 'dignity and respect'?

It is difficult to define either 'dignity' or 'respect' without using one of the terms to describe the other. Treating someone with respect is about ensuring their dignity. Ensuring that someone's dignity is protected involves treating them with respect.

A useful way to understand these concepts is to reflect on personal experience of them. We clearly know when we have been treated in a disrespectful way or placed in an undignified position (either in the physical or metaphorical sense). We feel it in a very powerful way.

Reflection point
> This reflection exercise is best done with a colleague. Think back to a situation where you have received healthcare, either as a patient or relative or as the informal carer of a patient, and have been treated in a way that you felt was disrespectful or undignified.

- Tell each other what happened.
- What did you feel at the time?

Perhaps you felt anger, embarrassment, hurt, sadness or a combination of these. Even thinking about the situation and the behaviour of the health professionals involved may bring back these feelings, perhaps many years after the actual event. This indicates how powerful these negative encounters can be and how they can live within people and colour future relationships with healthcare professionals.

Reflection point

Now think back to a situation where you have received healthcare and have been treated in a way that you felt was particularly respectful and where you felt measures were taken to maintain your dignity.

- How did it make you feel?

Usually people say it made them feel good and more inclined to be satisfied with the encounter. People are certainly aware when they have been treated with dignity and respect and often remember particular staff or teams for their skill in this aspect of care. When patients recount such situations they may use terms such as, 'They were really good'; 'They were kind and understanding'; 'They went out of their way to help me'.

- So what is it that makes such a difference to healthcare delivery? What is it that seems to be such a natural thing when we witness it, but is sadly so often missing in healthcare?

Reflection point

- What were the behaviours that were displayed in the two scenarios you identified above; the one where you were treated with dignity and respect, and the one where you were not?
- What did the health professionals do or say that contributed to your impression?

The constituent elements of dignity and respect that patients, carers and professionals identify (Walsh and Kowanko 2002; Whitehead and Wheeler 2008) include:

- being treated with empathy;
- being treated as an individual and not as a 'case', a 'number', an 'object' or a 'task';
- being treated with consideration, kindness, sympathy and compassion;
- having personal privacy protected and personal space respected;
- being given time;
- being listened to;
- being given explanations, choice and control;

- being kept informed;
- appropriate use of humour;
- absence of embarrassment.

The need to provide dignity and respect to patients and carers applies to everyone working in healthcare and this requirement is at the very core of nurses' professional code (NMC 2008). The elements of care listed above are reflected clearly in the *Code*, which states: 'The people in your care must be able to trust you with their health and wellbeing. To justify that trust, you must make the care of people your first concern, treating them as individuals and respecting their dignity'. The *Code* goes on to state that 'Failure to comply . . . may bring your fitness to practise into question and endanger your registration'.

Table 3.2 identifies some of the detail that the *Code* provides on the ways this should be demonstrated in nursing practice. It is clear that communication is the key to conveying the spirit of these principles in our work.

Table 3.2 Elements from the *Code*

Make the care of people your first concern, treating them as individuals and respecting their dignity

Treat people as individuals
- You must treat people as individuals and respect their dignity
- You must not discriminate in any way against those in your care
- You must treat people kindly and considerately
- You must act as an advocate for those in your care, helping them to access relevant health and social care, information and support

Respect people's confidentiality
- You must respect people's right to confidentiality
- You must ensure people are informed about how and why information is shared by those who will be providing their care
- You must disclose information if you believe someone may be at risk of harm, in line with the law of the country in which you are practising

Collaborate with those in your care
- You must listen to the people in your care and respond to their concerns and preferences
- You must support people in caring for themselves to improve and maintain their health
- You must recognize and respect the contribution that people make to their own care and wellbeing
- You must make arrangements to meet people's language and communication needs
- You must share with people, in a way they can understand, the information they want or need to know about their health

Ensure you gain consent
- You must ensure that you gain consent before you begin any treatment or care
- You must respect and support people's rights to accept or decline treatment and care
- You must uphold people's rights to be fully involved in decisions about their care
- You must be aware of the legislation regarding mental capacity, ensuring that people who lack capacity remain at the centre of decision-making and are fully safeguarded

---

Communicating dignity and respect verbally and non-verbally

Patients and carers must be able to trust that we are telling them the truth (see Chapter 9). Being honest with someone is a sign of respect for them as an individual with equal rights to oneself. This trust is built in a variety of ways and conveys the elements of care that go toward conferring dignity and respect through both verbal and non-verbal behaviour.

In terms of verbal communication it is obvious that what is said is important to people. Even where English is the common language between people, understanding cannot be taken for granted. The nursing and medical professions often use jargon, abbreviations and acronyms that are meaningless to service users and even to their colleagues in other departments. Whether this is done deliberately or not, it is excluding and undermines trust.

Patient perspective
'They stood in a huddle and discussed me just as if I wasn't there. I couldn't understand a word they were saying. It was complete gobbledegook to me!'

Activity
List the 10 most common acronyms and abbreviations used in your area of practice. For example, MSU (mid-stream sample of urine), TDS (three times a day). Show your non-nursing friends the list and ask them what the acronyms mean to them. In this way you will gain some idea of how poorly the general public understand nursing shorthand.

Activity
This activity is best undertaken with a group of colleagues.
Write down any abbreviations and acronyms you have come across and think of all the possible medical meanings for those abbreviations. To start you off, PND could mean:

• perinatal death;
• postnatal depression;
• paroxysmal nocturnal dyspnoea.

How would you feel if you were a patient and heard such an term used without knowing what it meant?

When people are on the receiving end of communication laden with jargon, abbreviations and acronyms that they don't understand it is likely to arouse a variety of emotions in them. In such situations people may feel angry, frustrated, confused, embarrassed, upset, humiliated, anxious, suspicious or any combination of these. Thus, it is important to ensure that we minimize the use of such terms or at least ensure that patients understand any technical language we or others are using in the course of their healthcare.

The range of non-verbal communication available is shown in Table 3.3. In most communication, the non-verbal part of the message is the one that is most attended to by the receiver. It is clear that how we say words and how people behave non-verbally during an encounter are the most powerful factors and deserve close attention (See Chapter 1).

Table 3.3 Elements of non-verbal communication

Paralinguistic factors – pitch, tone, rhythm, inflection, speed, volume, length of pauses before or within the communication

Eye contact or avoidance – duration of eye contact

Head movements – nodding, shaking

Facial expression – eyebrows, mouth

Posture – relaxed or tense, the direction of body lean, upright or slouched

Direction – facing toward or away from the other person

Touch – when, where, whether and how you touch

Distance between communicators – personal space

Activity

- How many ways can you say each of the following phrases?
  'That is really interesting'
  'Could you wait a moment please?'
  'I don't know'
- Vary the non-verbal aspects of your behaviour by using different tones, speeds and pitches. Combine these with combinations of different body language. For example, try different postures, gestures and facial expressions. You will find that you can communicate completely different attitudes, even while using the same words (patronizing, caring, intolerant, concerned and empathetic, dismissive, irritated, to name but a few). Try the combinations out on a colleague and see if they can guess the attitude behind the communication.

Listening

Arguably the most important of all the communication skills for conveying dignity and respect is that of listening. Patients and carers cannot be known as individuals if they are not listened to. Neither can their needs, hopes, fears or understanding of their situation be known. It is not only important to listen but it is also crucial that the person perceives that they are being listened to and this knowledge, in itself, is valued by service users as an indication of dignity and respect. The non-verbal communication skills that convey active listening are discussed more fully in Chapter 2.

Table 3.4 explains the way communication methods can be combined to either acknowledge someone positively or to reject them (negative acknowledgement).

Table 3.4 Positive and negative acknowledgement

- Positive acknowledgement involves the expression of warmth, equality and willingness to listen. We show we appreciate and understand the other person.
- Negative acknowledgement demonstrates coolness or rejection of the person. We show disrespect and rejection of the other person.

Positive acknowledging – making eye contact and smiling, open posture, listening, using encouraging non-verbal cues such as nodding, looking interested, open stance and gestures

Negative acknowledging – frowning or not making eye contact, turning away, looking bored or irritated, appearing not to listen by looking away or seeming distracted, closed stance

Activity

Sit in a waiting area of a hospital, clinic or GP surgery for half an hour and observe the communication between staff and patients.

- What non-verbal communication do you see?
- Is it congruent with what is being said?
- Do you see examples of positive and negative acknowledging?

You could record your observations and reflections on this exercise and put this in your portfolio of placement experience or CPD.

Non-verbal communication is so complex and used so naturally that little conscious attention is paid to the messages sent and received in this way. It is essential for nurses to develop skills to assess their own non-verbal communication. Self-awareness is the first step to improving the way in which dignity and respect are conveyed to patients and colleagues and is the basis for developing and communicating empathy for others.

Because healthcare professionals become so familiar with their own clinical areas, they may become desensitized to the environment and processes that take place as a matter of routine. It is much easier to observe in a different area because you see it with 'fresh eyes'. It can therefore be useful to undertake this exercise with a colleague from another clinical area, whose judgement you trust, and arrange to observe each other's area and exchange constructive feedback. Remember to note good practice as well as areas for improvement and to be aware that the feedback needs to be communicated in a way that is both useful and respectful. Feedback that is perceived as personal or blaming is unlikely to improve practice. There are some simple guidelines for the giving and receiving of feedback and these are discussed in Chapter 5. The important point is to critique the practice, not the person, and to discuss constructive ways forward.

Threats to good communication

There is evidence that patients and staff agree about the elements of care that communicate dignity and respect in healthcare. However, although both groups agree that it is important, it seems that staff may give it a lower priority (Elaswarapu 2007). It has been suggested that lack of interpersonal communication skills on the part of health professionals can be a problem (Walsh and Kowanko 2002). It also seems that there are times when even staff who possess these communication skills find they are likely to be compromised. The danger times are when interactions become routine and staff cease to see patients as individuals and more as a task in a long line of other tasks. Communication skills can also fail when staff are stressed or working under time pressures. There are so many competing demands on staff attention and targets to meet, that it is easy for them to lose sight of the way in which they are communicating. At these times it must be remembered that good communication skills conveying dignity and respect to patients and carers are not 'optional extras', but a fundamental and essential part of any healthcare professional's role.

The importance of empathy

Nurses need to try to see things from the patients' perspective. However, they also need to protect themselves from over-identification with their patient's situation, so that they remain in a position to help and support them rather than being overwhelmed by their problems. 'Put yourself in the patient's shoes but keep your socks on' is a useful mantra that is often repeated by health professionals in explaining empathy. However, trying to communicate empathy is not without its dangers. The worst outcome is for a patient to feel patronized. For example, the death of a parent will have a unique effect on each child left behind. Thus, saying to a recently bereaved child, 'I know exactly how you feel' can make the nurse appear insincere. It is often better to communicate empathy non-verbally and verbally reflect back to the individual the emotion that you can see in them; for example, 'I can see how devastated you are.'

It is essential for the nurse to understand the difference between empathy, sympathy and pity. It is easy to get pulled into a patient's distress, especially if the nurse has experienced, or is experiencing, a similar situation. These three emotions, pity, sympathy and empathy, can be summarized as follows (Wilmer 1968).

- Pity describes a relationship which separates physician and patient. Pity is often condescending and may entail feelings of contempt and rejection.
- Sympathy is when the physician experiences feelings as if he or she were the sufferer. Sympathy is thus shared suffering.
- Empathy is the feeling relationship in which the clinician understands the patient's plight as if the physician were the patient. The physician identifies with the patient and at the same time maintains a distance. Empathetic communication enhances the therapeutic effectiveness of the clinician–patient relationship.

Although Wilmer refers to physicians, these observations apply equally to all caring professionals including nurses.

Empathy helps determine the most considerate and compassionate way to behave towards the patient. We can anticipate situations that may cause distress, embarrassment and anxiety and take measures to avoid or at least ameliorate the effects. The ability to empathize is one of the attributes that patients value in nurses and it is only by actively listening to patients and being aware of both their verbal and non-verbal cues that we can understand their needs.

Below are two vignettes that are based on nursing situations that frequently occur. The activities based on them are designed to promote reflection on the part of the reader and may be used with colleagues to provoke discussion. The points raised after each activity are not exhaustive, but simply identify some important aspects for consideration.

Vignette   Visiting time

Mrs Garcia managed to get away from work early and rushed up to the hospital to be there within the appointed visiting time. She is there to see her mother who has recently been admitted to a medical ward. When she arrives at the ward there is a crowd of staff around the nurses' station. She is unsure what to do, so she hovers at the desk but nobody looks up. They all seem to be chatting or tapping away at computers. She coughs and moves forward to be noticed and one nurse glances up at her and then continues the conversation. Another person walks away and a third picks up the phone and starts a call.

- How do you think Mrs Garcia feels?

After a while Mrs Garcia says, 'Excuse me,' and a nurse looks up at her. 'I am here to see my mother, Mrs Grant.' The nurse sighs and continues to rifle through the pile of paper on the desk. 'She's not one of mine. Is she the COPD that came in today?' The nurse shouts up the corridor to another colleague 'Do we have a Mrs Grant?' 'Yes. The asthmatic in Bay 4,' comes the shouted reply. The nurse at the desk carries on with her paperwork and Mrs Garcia sets off up the corridor to find Bay 4.

- How is Mrs Garcia feeling now?

Activity

- Discuss or write down the ways in which the communication in the above vignette conveys a lack of respect and dignity for Mrs Garcia and her mother. How do the individual attitudes of the nurses contribute to such communication? How could the communication have been improved?
- What aspects of organizational culture lead to such poor communication and how can these be challenged and changed?

Below are some of the points that you may have identified from the last activity.

- There is no welcome for Mrs Garcia on the ward. A smile and a greeting from at least one member of staff would have helped to put her at ease.
- Mrs Garcia is already anxious and harassed and it is not clear who she should approach when she enters the ward. If there is no receptionist available, all staff should take responsibility for acknowledging visitors to the unit.
- Although Mrs Garcia indicates non-verbally that she needs help, nobody acknowledges her presence. Being sensitive to other people's non-verbal cues and responding appropriately to them is an important part of clinical practice.
- When Mrs Garcia finally speaks, the nurse indicates irritation by sighing. This indicates to Mrs Garcia that she is being a bother and is not really important enough to warrant disturbing the nurse. Suppressing the sigh and responding with a smile even though everyone is busy indicates to other people that they and their time is valuable and worthy of respect.
- By using the label of a medical diagnosis to identify Mrs Grant, it sounds as if her status as an individual is diminished. Is she just another asthmatic?
- Confidentiality is breached by shouting out the name, diagnosis and whereabouts of the patient for all to hear.
- Mrs Garcia is new to the environment. She is anxious and does not know where to find Bay 4. Anticipating this need by offering help, or better still providing a guide, would show empathy with her situation.

Vignette   A visit from the nurse

Mr McKay waits for the community nurse to call to change his leg dressing. He knows that she is due to visit today, but is not sure when. As he is hard of hearing he is afraid of missing the sound of the doorbell, so he has sat with the radio turned off all day. It takes him a long time to get to the front door, so he has also been worried about going up to the toilet or out to the back kitchen in case the nurse arrives while he is there.

When the nurse finally arrives he opens the door and lets her in. 'Hello Don. How are you? I'm here to do your dressing. Brrr it's cold outside.' The nurse bustles past him without waiting for an answer and is into the front room before Mr McKay can turn round. He is taken by surprise. This is a new nurse and they have never met before. Mr McKay starts the long journey back to his chair.

'I'll just pop and wash my hands. Is this the bathroom?' says the nurse cheerily, opening a broom cupboard. To Mr McKay's embarrassment the contents of the cupboard fall out all over the floor. By the time he gets back to his chair he finds the nurse has moved all the bits and bobs from his little side table and opened up a dressing pack on it. She is hovering with her gloved hands waiting. He wonders ruefully whether after this nurse has left he will be able to find the spectacles that had once been on the table.

- How do you think Mr McKay is feeling?

Activity

Identify the ways that the nurse's behaviour in this vignette conveys a lack of respect and dignity for Mr McKay. Why is the nurse behaving like this? How could this encounter have been improved?

Below are some of the points that you may have identified when working through the activity concerning Mr McKay's treatment.

- Pinpointing visit times is difficult, but giving Mr McKay an indication of when the visit will take place recognizes that his time is valuable too and that the business of his everyday life is not unimportant.
- The fact that the nurse did not introduce herself and her use of Mr McKay's first name without first asking his permission may be an attempt to be friendly and save time, but is rude.
- Barging into someone's house uninvited and/or entering a room uninvited is rude. Just because the nurse is there in a professional capacity does not make it less rude.
- Opening a door or cupboard in someone's house without asking permission led to Mr McKay feeling embarrassed. It shows a lack of empathy and a disregard for his feelings.
- Again the nurse may be saving time, but moving Mr McKay's belongings around without first asking permission demonstrates a particular lack of respect for his personal space.
- The nurse is disempowering Mr McKay by her behaviour and communication in this scenario. She is taking control and ownership of the space and setting the pace of the encounter to suit her busy schedule. She is not listening to Mr McKay even though she is in his home.

Respecting personal space, privacy and confidentiality

Everyone carries a sense of the personal space they occupy and control of that personal space is important to each person. Challenges to it or loss of control over it are stressful. If someone stands too close to a person in an everyday encounter, that person will feel uncomfortable and may unconsciously or consciously seek to increase the distance from the other person. The comfortable distance between people is usually determined by their relationship. In general, strangers are not tolerated to come as close as friends. The context of the encounter is also an influential factor in determining personal space. In a crowded tube train, people tolerate being very close to strangers in a way that they would not be comfortable with if the train were half empty. You may have noticed that people maintain their 'distance' or 'personal space' despite the close proximity of others, by avoiding eye contact with each other. As soon as the crowd diminishes, people move into a space to re-establish a comfortable personal distance. There are many factors that influence the personal space we feel comfortable with. For example the age, gender, cultural background and personal relationship of the people involved and our professional relationship with them.

Nurses, by virtue of their professional status, have the privilege of being allowed into an individual's personal space to carry out personal care or procedures. However, consent to do so should be sought from the patient on every occasion. Just because an element of care has been carried out on one day does not mean that you have the patient's permission to do so again without asking.

Personal space can also be considered in terms of the territory around us that we lay claim to as 'ours'. Mr McKay's vignette demonstrates that nurses working within the service user's home can forget that they are in the patient's territory and for nurses working in hospital settings this can be even more of a problem. Nurses are inclined to consider the whole of a ward or department space as their own territory, while a patient, once allocated to a bed or a chair space, considers the space around them as their own.

Reflection point

Imagine you are at a meeting or at a table for group work. You have arrived early and set your papers out in front of you.

- Another person arrives a bit later, sits on the chair next to yours, even though most of the others are empty, and spreads their papers out so that they are nearly on top of yours.
- How would feel? Would you do anything and if so why?

If we go back to consider the patient claiming the bed space as their own, they may feel similar unease if nurses continue to treat the space as theirs. Nurses should signal their respect for the patient's personal space by gaining consent before entering into the curtained bed space. Mr McKay found that the nurse had claimed his home as her own space and moved around, opened doors and rearranged things, presumably oblivious to the discomfort she was causing him.

As demonstrated above, privacy is linked to personal space and modesty is a similarly related concept. Privacy and modesty are often interlinked in that we may have to provide privacy to protect someone's modesty. Privacy of the body is an important aspect of communicating dignity and respect, and nurses need to take steps to protect a patient's modesty. In taking such action nurses communicate to patients that they empathize with their feelings of potential embarrassment or fear of exposure and respect them enough to take steps to avoid or ameliorate situations that may engender such feelings.

Activity

What steps would you take to protect the patient's privacy and modesty in the following situations? How would you intervene to avoid the patient being embarrassed? Make notes of your own ideas on each scenario and then share these with colleagues in order to discuss possible options and contingencies.

1 A patient with an indwelling urinary catheter and drainage bag and wearing a nightie needs to be wheeled on a trolley to the X-ray department.
2 A patient on bed rest wears dentures but doesn't want anyone else to know. She has told you that she needs to clean them.
3 A patient in a clinic consulting room has to get undressed and wait for a doctor to come and examine them.
4 A young woman approaches the reception desk at a GP surgery wanting to ask for emergency contraception.

Below are just some points that you may have considered.

Situation 1

- Offering a dressing gown or covering the patient with a blanket. Making sure it is big enough to enable the patient to cover themselves from chin to toe if they choose to do so.
- Covering the catheter drainage bag to prevent the urine being on display.
- Adjusting the trolley so that the patient may sit up rather than lying flat, which is less dignified (if safe to do so).
- Ensuring that the patient's notes are covered if the trolley is wheeled through public areas.

Situation 2

- Asking the patient discreetly whether they would prefer to clean the dentures themselves or whether they would like you to do it.
- If they want to do it themselves, providing the equipment for them to do so and if possible leaving them alone until they have finished the task and replaced the dentures.
- Ensuring that the patient feels secure and knows that no one will interrupt the procedure by coming unexpectedly through the bed curtains. For example, by using privacy pegs to hold the curtains together and to signal that people should seek permission from the patient within before opening them.

Situation 3

- Be clear in communicating to them how far they need to undress for the examination.
- Ensure the patient has a private space in which to undress.
- Provide and point out to the patient adequate covering for them (gown or blanket) when they are undressed.

- Ensure the patient cannot be seen from the corridor when the door to the room is opened.
- Ensure the patient knows they will not be interrupted while they are changing and how to indicate when they are ready.
- Ensure the room is marked 'engaged' and that anyone entering the room knocks first and waits for an answer.

Situation 4

- Ensure a queuing system is in place that reduces the chance of others in the queue overhearing conversations with staff at the desk.
- Be alert to non-verbal and verbal cues from the patient that they are embarrassed or uncomfortable in stating their reason for attending. Act to provide a private place for the conversation to take place.
- Be discreet. Moderate the voice and avoid being explicit about the reason for attendance if the conversation is at risk of being overheard.
- Ensure that any medication prescribed is handed to the patient in non-transparent bags to avoid bystanders being able to see the nature of the pre-scription.

In the examples given above, it is clear that ensuring privacy often depends on communication both with colleagues and the patient. You may notice that in these scenarios, as in most nursing situations, informing the patient about what is about to happen and offering them choice is desirable. Where control over an experience or a situation is not possible for patients, then providing the opportunity for them to be able to predict what will happen is the next best option.

In a similar way, privacy is also related to confidentiality. The legal requirements on healthcare professionals to ensure appropriate confidentiality with regard to patient information is discussed in Chapter 9, but the link between privacy, confidentiality and communicating dignity and respect is worth reflecting on.

Reflection point

Patient privacy and confidentiality are endangered in the following situations. How should you act to protect them?

- You are at the patient's bedside and they wish to discuss something personal with you, but there is only a curtain between you and the patient in the next bed.
- You are taking a meal break with a colleague in the hospital canteen and they begin to discuss one of the patients in your care.

Humour in communication dignity and respect

It is clear that communicating in a way that conveys dignity and respect and takes into account an individual's personal space and privacy is a serious business, but we all know that humour can be a wonderful tool in aiding such communication. It can relieve a stressful or embarrassing situation, help build a therapeutic relationship and equalize the power in a patient – professional interaction as you laugh together. *However*, humour is a double-edged sword and it is worth considering the ways in which it can be used to either promote dignity and respect or undermine them. For example:

- Laughing *at* someone can humiliate and demean them.
- Laughing *with* someone can help to equalize the power relationship in a situation and empower the service user.
- Laughing over someone or excluding someone from a shared joke can be hurtful and disempowering.
- Cruel or deliberately demeaning humour, such as sarcasm, has no place in professional practice.
- The mood of the patient and the situation need to be judged carefully – are they in the mood for a joke? Is the situation appropriate for you to introduce humour?
- Responding positively to a patient's humour helps build a relationship and is an opportunity for them to show their individual personality and be acknowledged as an individual.
- In many situations humour can relieve stress and embarrassment but in others it can create it.
- Humour may be used to hide true feelings of fear, anxiety or embarrassment. This is true for both the nurse and the patient.

There are no hard and fast rules for using humour to communicate dignity and respect but it is wise to be cautious and gentle with humour. What one patient finds funny may be offensive to another and while the same patient may be open to humour in one situation, they may feel it is inappropriate in another. Therefore, being sensitive to the verbal and non-verbal cues they offer is the only answer and taking the lead from the patient is safest when making judgements as to whether humour is appropriate.

Stereotyping and labelling: the enemies of dignity and respect

Treating people and communicating with them as individuals in their own right is at the heart of providing dignified and respectful care. Communicating recognition of that individuality means that there is a need to recognize any prejudices that nurses may have and work to eliminate them. Stereotypes are widely-shared generalizations about members of a social group and these generalizations are highly simplified, often derogatory and often associated with prejudice. They may be based on, and lead to, ageism, sexism, racism or other kinds of negative discriminatory attitudes and behaviours. Many prejudices are deeply rooted and not always amenable to eradication by rational argument, and particularly where this is the case, nurses need to guard against acting on them. To do so would lead to discriminatory behaviour, which is both against the law and in violation of the NMC *Code* (2008).

The reader may wish to refer to The Equality and Human Rights Commission, established in 2007, which provides a useful source of information. Its aim is to end discrimination and harassment of people due to disability, age, religion or belief, race, gender or sexual orientation (see www.equalityhumanrights.com).

Patient perspective

'I could tell by her attitude that as soon as the practice nurse looked at my notes and saw that I was only 17 years old, she thought "another teenage mother" and from that moment on she assumed I was a waste of space and would be a rotten mum.'

Health professionals constantly need to communicate with each other about the patients in their care. Although such communication, both oral and written, is vital, it can also be a vehicle for passing on stereotypes and prejudices. By listening to handovers or communications between health professionals you may come across the use of stereotypes and 'labels' for particular groups or so-called 'types' of patient. This is a shorthand that professionals may slip into, often without any ill intent. However, these labels can lead to inequalities in service and care. For example, professionals may carelessly use labels such as 'bedblocker', 'difficult patient', ' old dear' or 'timewaster', and anyone unfortunate enough to be given such a label may be treated in accordance with the label as opposed to their own individual needs and personality. If part of being treated with dignity is to be treated as an individual, then acting on the assumptions that accompany stereotyping and labelling may achieve the opposite.

Reflection point

- What are the labels that are sometimes used when describing patients or relatives in your clinical arena?
- How are they used?
- What assumptions do they lead to?
- Do the labels predispose the patients to different levels of care?

One example of a negative stereotype associated with older people is the view that they are all confused, vulnerable, childlike and needy. These attributes may be true of some individuals (of any age), but to apply this stereotype means that all older people are assumed to have these characteristics and are approached in a way that is both inappropriate and condescending. Sometimes stereotypes will pop into our heads and it would be foolish to claim that they never do, but we can and should make concerted efforts to reject them and ensure that practice is never based on them.

Conclusion

It is essential that we think about patients and how healthcare professionals regard and treat them. People become patients, but still remain people throughout their journey with disease and illness towards health or death. Patients need to be regarded as fellow human beings rather than simply 'someone with a medical problem'. There are a number of points that are important to remember when caring for people:

- Health professionals need to communicate in ways that convey that they value the patient or carer as an individual person who deserves to be treated with dignity and respect, and to do this even in the most difficult and trying circumstances.
- It is essential for nurses to develop skills to assess their own verbal and non-verbal communication. Self-awareness is the first step to improving the way in which we convey dignity and respect to patients and colleagues and is the basis for developing and communicating empathy for others.
- Communicating dignity and respect must include consideration for the patient's personal space, privacy and their right to confidentiality.
- Listening and being sensitive to the verbal and non-verbal cues offered by patients and carers is crucial in conveying dignity and respect.
- Humour can be a wonderful aid to communication but it can also be dangerous. Taking the lead from the patient is safest when making judgements as to whether humour is appropriate.
- As an important part of being treated with dignity is to be treated as an individual, the assumptions that accompany stereotyping and labelling other people are to be avoided at all costs.

References

DH (Department of Health) (2003) *The Essence of Care: Patient-focused Benchmarking for Health Care Practitioners*. London: DH.

Elaswarapu, R. (2007) Dignity in care for older people in hospital – measuring what matters, *Working with Older People*, 1(2): 15–19.

NMC (Nursing and Midwifery Council) (2008) *The Code: Standards of Conduct, Performance and Ethics for Nurses and Midwives*, www.nmc-uk.org.uk (accessed 11 March 2010).

Walsh, K. and Kowanko, I. (2002) Nurses' and patients' perceptions of dignity, *International Journal of Nursing Practice*, 8: 143–51.

Whitehead, J. and Wheeler, H. (2008) Patients' experience of privacy and dignity, Part 2: an empirical study, *British Journal of Nursing*, 7(7): 458–64.

Wilmer, H.A. (1968) The doctor-patient relationship and issues of pity, sympathy and empathy, *British Journal of Medical Psychology*, 41(3): 243–8.

4 Using technology to communicate

Sarah Kraszewski

This chapter explores the issues concerning effective communication using technology. It includes exploration of synchronous and asynchronous means of communication, the use of mobile devices and the use of technology to facilitate the delivery of healthcare. Examples and episodes of care are included to encourage reflection upon the use and impact of technology on the lives of patients and professionals.

Learning outcomes

By the end of this chapter you should be able to:
1 Recognize the importance of using information technology (IT) in modern healthcare.
2 Learn how to communicate appropriately using the telephone and email.
3 Understand the use and abuse of mobile electronic devices.
4 Understand how to use the internet as an effective learning resource.

Introduction

Developments in IT in recent years have exerted an extensive and complex influence on the ways in which human beings interact with each other, from both a personal and professional perspective. There are many ways to connect us together. Modern healthcare depends upon communicating information and requires nurses to develop and refine their communication skills using technology. Information needs to be collected and utilized in reliable and robust formats to enable safe and effective usage. Access to patients and other healthcare staff can be facilitated face to face, but also via technology such as the telephone and email. A bewildering array of websites is available to access information on any given symptom or illness and patients may often arrive armed with their research and their interpretation of a diagnosis. This makes the skill of communicating via technologies and the dexterity of finding and using evidence-based resources essential for the nurse. This chapter aims to highlight the skills needed to support effective care utilizing commonly available communication technologies and to provide a brief overview of the national programme for information technology, 'Connecting for Health'.

Communicating using technology

The advent of the IT age has enabled the delivery of healthcare to be supported by technology across a variety of locations and circumstances. The interactive possibilities of computers and the internet have influenced this development and can offer a rich source of information and interactivity, without individuals needing to travel for a face-to-face encounter. Use of technologies such as email or teleconferencing can facilitate interactivity between two or more individuals, saving time, cost of the journey and the environmental impact of travel. It can also provide flexibility and facilitate home working. However, this is not without its limitations or costs. Gore *et al.* (2002: 848) suggest that the development of these technologies has contributed to 'boundaryless lives', in that the new technologies demand a workforce that can be 'flexible and adaptive', which may lead to a blurring of the boundaries between home and work. This can 'increase and intensify the demands made upon people in their everyday lives, speeding up the pace of their lives and requiring the increased micro-management and multi-tasking of daily experiences' (Bull 2007: 72). Additionally, the speed of communication available may not necessarily lead to improved communication (Robb 2004). Successful communication requires interactivity on a number of levels. It may occur face to face, via printed materials or through the use of technology. Interactivity is a two-way process, providing a channel for response and feedback.

> **Vignette   Work–life balance**
> Obusola works in a managerial role for a large healthcare organization and is able to access her email account and the organization's network from home. She enjoys the convenience of being able to work from home, saving the time and expense of travel. She gets up early and sometimes goes straight to the computer in her dressing gown and before she knows it lunchtime has arrived and she isn't even dressed. Obusola feels the boundaries between her working life and home life are getting rather blurred.

Obusola's situation is becoming more common as technology permits remote access and removes the physical boundaries of the working environment. An individual can easily slip into a situation where work obscures home life and find themselves working much longer hours. Although the flexibility is an advantage, it is important that Obusola exerts control and inserts structure into her day to ensure effective time management and a healthy work–life balance.

Synchronous and asynchronous communication

Communication may be described as *synchronous* (both parties participate at the same time) – for example, when using the telephone or an internet chat room; alternatively it may be *asynchronous* (the communication may take place over a longer period of time, with participants not necessarily participating at the same time) – for example, when using email or a bulletin board. There are advantages and disadvantages that apply to both situations.

Activity

- Make a list of the different activities that can be undertaken using the internet or telephone in both healthcare and everyday life – for example, shopping, banking. What is the impact of not being able to see or hear the person you are interacting with?
- Review the following types of encounters you will have with patients, staff and relatives and write down the advantages and disadvantages of using different media to communicate. An example has been completed.

Type of encounter

1 Telephone

- Advantages: technology widely available, instant access to health professional, auditory cues.
- Disadvantages: confidentiality – ensuring the caller is who they say they are, no visual cues, expectation of an instant response.

2 Face to face
3 Letter
4 Message book
5 Fax machine
6 Teleconference
7 Video conference
8 SMS text
9 Smart phone
10 Email
11 Bulletin-board discussion
12 Social networking site
13 Instant internet chat facility

Synchronous communication, such as participating in a telephone call, is quick, offering the opportunity for an instant response in time and place. It offers the potential of a speedy, instantaneous response to a request and can be a satisfying experience for both parties. Conversely, the expectation of an instant response may cause stress for one or both parties. It may not be possible to provide that instant response if one party needs to consult with a third. It does not allow time for either party to reflect or think about a response for any length of time. Telephone calls may be recorded (e.g. by NHS Direct), but this may not be routinely in place, which raises implications for the accuracy of record-keeping.

Activity

A patient telephones the ward asking your advice regarding their abdominal scar from recent surgery.

- What information do you require to make an assessment and how would you advise the patient?
- How would you record your telephone conversation?
- What advantages or disadvantages does the telephone impose on this situation?

Asynchronous communication, such as engaging in an email message, although slower, allows all parties the opportunity to reflect upon and consider their response, to access advice from other parties without 'loss of the moment', before replying. If using a text-based medium, an electronic copy of the communication is automatically generated, providing a record. In some respects this may be considered a more effective means of communication, but each technology used has to be considered in the light of its purpose.

Commonly-used technologies

The telephone

The most commonly used and familiar technology is the telephone. It is available as landlines and mobile devices. Communication devices (such as 'smart phones') have evolved to provide internet services as well as telephone communication. Many health professionals are now being equipped with mobile devices to enable them to be constantly in touch and available.

Reflection point
- The use of technology encourages a 24-hour, seven days a week assumption of availability. Consider the impact of this from a personal and professional context.
- Is this a positive use of the technology or does it encourage unrealistic expectations and demands on the individual's time?

Telephone skills

Developing appropriate telephone skills is an important aspect of nursing. In all settings many communications will occur using the telephone, such as relatives making enquiries, taking results over the telephone or making calls to other departments. The way in which the telephone is answered in a professional context is different to the way it might be answered at home. When answering the telephone, you should always clearly state your location, status and name in a confident manner. It is important to be aware of the loss of visual cues in a telephone call and to recognize the finer cues regarding subtlety of speech, pauses, breathlessness and other non-visual cues that may provide information about the caller or give the caller information about you (Sully and Dallas 2005). The call should have a structure. There should be a logical beginning (signalled by the way you answer) and a defined end (Bishop 2008).

Vignette   Breathless

Julie is working in the GP surgery when a patient, Mrs Patel, rings for advice. She has a history of asthma and is on regular medication. She is worried as she has been feeling more breathless and has needed to use her reliever medication more frequently over the last couple of days. As Julie talks to Mrs Patel she becomes aware that she can hear Mrs Patel's breathing on the telephone and notes that she is unable to finish her sentences in one breath. She enquires regarding Mrs Patel's peak expiratory flow rate and is informed that it is 350l/m. Julie is aware that there are limitations to telephone consultations and it is not possible to diagnose over the telephone. However, she can make an assessment and decides that Mrs Patel would benefit from coming to the surgery to see the nurse for assessment of her asthma.

The observation made by Julie provided an added facet to the assessment that would not have been possible in an email or textual communication.

Reflection point

Think about how you communicate by telephone with patients.

- What are the advantages and disadvantages for both the nurse and the caller?
- Discuss this with colleagues in the clinical environment and find out their perspective.

Confidentiality

Confidentiality issues must be considered when using the telephone. A telephone call taken in the middle of a ward, office or waiting room may lead to a loss of confidentiality. Care must be taken to ensure privacy and to avoid confidential information being overheard. It may be necessary to take the call in a private room, close the door or lower your voice. Many calls will relate directly to imparting and receiving information about patients and it is imperative that when any information is given out that you are sure of the identity of the caller and whether it is appropriate to give them the information (Sully and Dallas 2005). If necessary, look up the caller's details and ring them back.

Activity

Tanya is a patient on the ward and has undergone gynaecological surgery on the morning list. She has not yet sufficiently recovered from the anaesthetic to have the details of her surgery discussed with her. Her husband Greg telephones the ward and you answer the telephone. Greg asks how his wife is and then proceeds to ask for details of the surgery.

- How do you respond?
- Consider how you would uphold Tanya's confidentiality while maintaining a constructive dialogue with her husband.

You may wish to consider:

- The NMC (2008) *Code*.
- Who the caller is.
- The privacy and confidentiality of the patient.
- The Caldicott principles, which resulted from the Caldicott Report of 1997 regarding how patient information was used and managed in a healthcare setting. The 'Caldicott Guardian' can advise on confidentiality and the management of patient information in the clinical setting (DH 2010).

Mobile devices

Many nurses are now equipped with mobile devices to aid communication in the work context. In modern living, almost every space has been colonized by the mobile phone (Bull 2007). We will all have had the experience of hearing one end of somebody's conversation and calls undertaken can become both private and public. This highlights the fact that for the health professional, care should be exercised when using a mobile phone as there is the potential to breach confidentiality. Additionally, having a mobile phone can make the user easily accessible to the whole world. There may be a sense of total availability, and for an individual to be controlled by others in an 'anytime, anywhere' fashion. This can lead to interruptions, increasing social demands and blurring boundaries between work and leisure, leading to stress (De Gornay 2002, cited by Bull 2007: 68). Mobile phones can enable users to change plans quickly, micro-managing their time, and have become an everyday tool in modern life (Robb 2004). It can be a frustrating and annoying experience for those in the company of someone who is frequently answering or checking their mobile phone. However, the mobile phone user can exert some control in such situations and ensure that the phone is turned on only when appropriate, and switched to voicemail when it is not or at least set to silent or vibrate. The voicemail facility allows the user to respond to a contact at a convenient and appropriate time, however, the mobile phone user may experience feelings of guilt or stress as a result of an unanswered call and it requires planning to find a suitable time to return the call, or there may not be time to return the call, which in itself can increase the feelings of guilt and stress.

Reflection point

Over the next few days, at both home and work, think about how, where and when you use your mobile phone.

- Consider its impact on other people and the situations where you choose to use it.
- Note how you feel when you have missed a call or are unable to reach the person who left you a message.

Vignette   Overheard conversations

Mr Zebrowski is an elderly man living in his own home. He receives visits from the community nursing team to dress his leg ulcer. The district nurse, Claudette, has been provided with a mobile phone to enable her to keep contact with the community nursing team, and also to make and receive calls from patients on her caseload. As she arrives in Mr Zebrowski's home, her mobile rings and she decides to answer it. The call is from the family of another patient on her caseload and she proceeds to hold a detailed discussion regarding that patient's care, while in Mr Zebrowski's home. As she ends the call, Mr Zebrowski asks if that was his friend George she was discussing, whom he knows receives visits from the same community nursing team.

By answering the call in the patient's home, Claudette compromised the confidentiality of another patient, and also demonstrated a lack of respect regarding the privilege of being a guest in the home of Mr Zebrowski. If the call was urgent it would have been more appropriate to return to her car for the conversation, or the phone should be turned to silent while in a patient's home.

Vignette   New text message

Student Nurse Gosling is accompanying the community nursing team as part of his community semester. With the community staff nurse, Staff Nurse Turay, he visits the home of Mr James, a patient with multiple sclerosis who has limited mobility and requires care that the community nurse provides while the student observes. Student Nurse Gosling feels like a spare part and his attention starts to wander. His mobile phone is switched to silent/vibrate and he notices he has received a text message. He chooses to read and answer the text message. Staff Nurse Turay glares at him and asks him to pay attention.

- Imagine you are Staff Nurse Turay and are supervising Student Nurse Gosling. Explain to Student Nurse Gosling why the use of his personal mobile phone is inappropriate and unprofessional while on duty in a patient's home.
- Suggest ways in which Staff Nurse Turay could avoid this happening in the future.

Patient perspective

'I've had the nurse coming to see me for a long time – we know each other well and I look forward to seeing her. She always treats me and my home with respect. I couldn't believe what I was seeing when the nurse she brought along to learn was fiddling with his phone. These youngsters have no respect.'

Mobile phones can also be used as a surveillance tool, offering both positive and negative attributes. They can be used to check someone's whereabouts. A parent may ring their child to check they are safe, a son may provide his elderly mother with a mobile phone to maintain contact from anywhere. Use of a mobile phone may form part of a 'lone worker' policy: community health professionals may ring their base before entering a particular person's home, there may be codes to indicate there is a problem (e.g. ringing the office for the 'yellow file' which may be a code for assistance required) and they may text or ring on leaving the premises to confirm they are on their way back to base or a subsequent appointment.

Short messaging service (SMS) texting is a more discreet and less intrusive medium provided by the mobile phone. Its use should be carefully selected. There are circumstances where a telephone call might resolve an issue more quickly. Texting has been incorporated into healthcare through the use of SMS texts to communicate with service users and may also be used by healthcare workers to communicate with each other.

Vignette   Receiving results

Angela attended a sexual health clinic and was offered a chlamydia screening test from the National Chlamydia Screening Programme. She undertook the test and completed the form to indicate how she would like to be notified of the result. She was offered the option of receiving the results by text message (SMS), telephone call, email or by post. She ticked the box to indicate she would prefer her results by SMS. She received a text two weeks later advising her that her test was negative. Using SMS to notify results provides a discreet, economic, accessible and convenient means to communicate screening test results to suitable groups of patients.

Patient perspective

'Getting my result by text suited me – it was quicker and more convenient as it won't get lost in the post, and I didn't have to remember to go and collect post as it came straight to my phone. It also meant that no one else would be able to read it.'

(Angela, age 19)

Email

Email is being used extensively as a means of communication, both between health professionals and between health professionals and patients. There are services on the internet that offer the latest information via email bulletins (e.g. those from the National Prescribing Centre) and many sites offer evidence-based guidelines and reviews. In an age where it is the norm to use internet services for shopping and banking, health professionals need to become proficient in using these media to improve the efficiency of communication in healthcare.

Email provides a convenient asynchronous means of communication in both home and work environments. Many people now have a home and/or work email address. Every NHS employee has access to an email account via their organization's network, offering functions beyond the capability to send and receive emails, such as calendars, meeting requests, task lists and other management tools aimed at supporting the organization of time and work (Tyrrell 2002). NHS staff may also set up an NHS net account, which permits remote access to email. As with other technologies, email offers advantages and disadvantages. Using it allows the user to send a written communication to the recipient, who will read and respond at a time convenient to them. It is cheaper, faster, more convenient and less obtrusive than a phone call. As an asynchronous medium it allows time to consider and reflect upon a response. It provides a written record of the communication, enhancing record-keeping.

However, caution should be observed. The writer or responder should take care when composing their communication as it could be misinterpreted without the visual or auditory cues afforded by body language, facial expressions, tone and volume that accompany a face-to-face encounter. The use of wit, irony and sarcasm need to be managed with great care to avoid offence. There is the possibility of an email being sent to the wrong recipient or that the recipient may forward it on to a wider audience that the original sender may not have intended to share the message with. There may be a 'trail' of messages on the email not intended for the current recipient or someone may have used a different email to send you something that contains inappropriate matter in the forwarded email.

Email is certainly an extremely useful tool in the modern business environment. To utilize it effectively is a skill in itself and it is important to develop strategies to manage email, rather than letting it manage you. Personal and business accounts may be managed together or separately depending upon an individual's prefer-ence and governance issues in the organization. All healthcare organizations have an 'acceptable use' policy for email and IT systems and it is essential to familiar-ize yourself with it to avoid the potential for disciplinary action following abuse of the system. Such policies are necessary as the employing organization may be held responsible for employees' actions when using the system – for example, if a potentially libellous email is sent, which might result in litigation (Lilley 2006).

The use of the preview panes, spam filters and a good filing system can make email manageable. Responses in a work environment need to be short, polite and focused. Remember that email lacks the subtlety of voice or body language and never send 'flaming' messages (ones that are rude or angry). An unfortunate choice of words, capital letters or punctuation can alter the interpretation of a message, which may then inadvertently cause at best a misunderstanding, and at worst offence, leading to litigation. If you receive a rude or angry email, wait a while before responding, so you avoid reacting in the heat of the moment. Indiscriminate use of the 'reply all' option should be discouraged as this catches others up in the responses unnecessarily, overloading their inboxes, and hence using valuable time to sort through the messages.

There are adaptations to support text-based electronic communication, which utilize a series of symbols and customs to denote expressions (such as smileys, shocked faces and winks), the use of which aims to enrich communication in this dimension. Many examples can be found on the internet and some are shown below.

:)	Smiley face
:D	Very smiley face
:(	Sad face
;)	Wink
:p	Joking face
:o!	Shocked face
:s	Confused face

However, 'emoticons' may not be appropriate for use in formal email communications within an organization and are better reserved for personal and social use.

Reflection point
- Think about how you compose emails to others.
- Consider the different approaches you need to take when communicating with friends and when communicating with colleagues, other services and patients.

Activity
Read the emails below.

Dear All,
I'm trying to get the policy written for wound care and despite sending it out several times no-ones bothered to respond. I feel like a lone worker here! Is anyone going to contribute?‽?

Cheers couch potatoes!
Jean

dear sir,
im very interested in the job u advertised and have attached my cv look forward to hearing from you
jane smith

hi george
nice TO MEEt you the othe r day. Can u send me a list of akll the relevant contacTS PLEaseso I can follop up
manty tjanks
saraH

- How would you feel if you received any of the above emails?
- What impressions do you form about the people sending them?
- Over the next few days sort your emails into those you consider to be well written and those that have provoked negative feelings.
- What are the characteristics of these communications that made you react positively or negatively?

Useful advice on the effective use of email can be found at www.liv.ac.uk/csd/email/emailuse.htm (University of Liverpool 2009).

Using the internet: staff and patients

The internet is an enormous unregulated mass of information, with much of it available to anyone. The world is out there and accessible at the click of a mouse. It is an area with few rules, individuals are able to express themselves freely and everyone else can read it (Zittrain 2008). This provides many advantages in terms of being able to access information without moving from the computer and it allows connectivity between people and organizations. For the nurse it provides easy access to a range of resources that can support professional development and enhance patient care. However, there is a skill in selecting resources that are evidence-based and rejecting those that are based on conjecture, opinion and hearsay. As a health professional, there will be access via the NHS system to decision-making software and evidenced-based resources. The Clinical Knowledge Summaries (CKS) from the National Electronic Library for Health (NELH) and available to all on the web, are particularly useful for both nurses and patients.

Service users may frequently arrive armed with their internet research on their disease or condition and expect the nurse to be able to comment upon it. It is important to familiarize yourself with a publicly available range of resources to recommend to patients. Examples of this include the NHS immunization website, CKS and the NHS stop smoking website. 'Athens' is a controlled password system that allows secure login and access to online subscription resources. NHS and educational organizations offer access to employees and students, enabling health professionals to search for evidence-based resources via a number of databases and to utilize search strategies to locate information and research from reliable sources.

Internet security

Security measures must be in place when accessing and using the internet. There are many hostile interlopers in the form of spyware and viruses. The storage of information and access to that information must be robust and in line with data protection legislation. It has become a regular feature of the news that a laptop, data stick or CD-ROM containing confidential information has been lost or stolen.

Data protection

The Data Protection Act (1998) affects the use of computers and management of the information stored upon them. It is a complex area of legislation which is encapsulated into eight principles. Personal data must be:

- fairly and lawfully processed;
- processed for limited purposes;
- adequate, relevant and not excessive;
- accurate;
- not kept longer than necessary;
- processed in accordance with the data subjects' rights;
- secure;
- not transferred to countries without adequate protection.

Within the NHS, patient information is an obvious concern, but data protection also affects employees' information, and other areas where data may be managed and stored (see Chapter 9).

Communicating with the world via the internet is becoming an everyday part of our lives and includes social networking sites and areas such as YouTube, which enables one to communicate with many people quickly and easily. 'Netiquette' is a term used to describe a 'code of conduct' for appropriate behaviour when communicating via the internet and it is useful to be mindful of these principles when using the web in either a professional or personal context. A number of guides are readily available, for example 'Netiquette' held at www.albion.com/netiquette/corerules.html (Shea 2004). It is also important to remember that nurses are bound by their professional code of conduct (NMC 2008) and should exercise discretion when using internet-based communication (such as participating in social networking sites) as some behaviour or comments may contravene the *Code* or violate contractual agreements. There are reports of nurses being disciplined for inappropriate use of NHS Trust resources when inappropriate internet activity has been undertaken during working hours, or for criticizing employers on such sites (Reymond 2008; *Nursing Standard* 2009).

Selecting an appropriate medium to communicate

When choosing to communicate, it is necessary to consider which technology is the most appropriate to use. There are a number of issues that need to be taken into account. In brief, these may be summarized into three components:

- Who is the recipient of the communication?
- What is the purpose of the communication?
- Can the recipient access the message?

To expand this further, the 'who' aspect requires consideration of the detail concerning the communication. Will this communication be with an individual (one to one) or with a group (one to many)? A number of technologies can be used either way – teleconferencing can be used to facilitate a group discussion and an email can be used as a one to many medium. Likewise a video conference might be considered. Using these tools enables people to communicate remotely without time and money spent travelling, but may enable them to see each other and so pick up some of the visual cues afforded by face-to-face communication. Further influence emanates from whether this is a formal or informal communication and deliberation on the purpose. Is this a communication to a group of colleagues, contacting a patient, or a chat with a friend? If this is a formal communication in the work environment to colleagues or to a patient, have governance issues been considered? Does it adhere to the policies and guidelines that support governance? IT systems in the NHS have security protocols which may block certain email addresses to protect against 'spam' (the use of mass emailing to send unsolicited messages). Are there guidelines regarding the content of emails, the type of attachments that may be sent and the footers that must be used? Can the person or group you are communicating with access the same technology that you are using? Is your computer software compatible with others?

Vignette   Cannot open the file

Danny, a nurse lecturer, was sent a flyer by one of his ex-students advertising a study day being held in the student's workplace. The student asked Danny to forward the flyer to colleagues in the university and practice areas to publicize it. When Danny attempted to open it, the attachment was in a non-standard file type so he was unable gain access. Unfortunately neither could any colleagues so the message was lost.

Reflection point
- Have you experienced something similar to Danny's problem? What were the consequences and how did you feel?
- When you send a message, does the recipient have the correct skills and equipment to be able to access it?
- Do they have any special needs (such as visual or hearing impairment) that will make one medium more appropriate than another?

Taking these issues into account will assist selection of the most appropriate medium for the communication and will help to ensure successful receipt of the message. For example, a tutor may select a virtual learning environment to share a PowerPoint presentation with students, a manager needing to circulate a safety alert may use an email group, and wider dissemination may be achieved by using a web page or medium such as YouTube.

NHS Connecting for Health

Healthcare organizations have complex communication needs, both within an individual organization and when interacting with other organizations. Using IT in healthcare has clear benefits for patient safety by providing structured care, highlighting errors and providing evidence-based decision support tools at the point of care delivery (Bates and Gawande 2003).

The delivery of healthcare is undergoing transformation by the integration of IT in enhancing and promoting communication between health workers and patients. 'Connecting for Health', the national programme for IT, is possibly the largest and most ambitious system ever attempted. The project commenced in April 2005 to integrate communication technology into the NHS and provide a twenty-first-century service. It aims to provide lifelong electronic patient records (EPRs), online access to patient records by clinicians, where and when they need them (across organizational boundaries) and evidence-based information to clinicians. Additionally, other innovations such as electronic booking and prescription services are integrated into the system.

Connecting for Health has been subject to adverse publicity as costs are rumoured to have escalated and implementation has exceeded the original timeline. However, for all the reported difficulties, it has introduced many benefits for patients and practitioners by enhancing communication, improving access to care and managing information effectively and efficiently. Evidently it is necessary for all staff working in the NHS in both clinical and administrative roles to develop effective communication skills using IT.

Reflection point
Think about your own IT skills.

- Are they sufficient to interact effectively with the technology or are there training needs to add to your personal development plan?
- Are you aware of how to access IT training provided by your organization?

The implementation of EPRs has required changes in working practices. EPRs offer many benefits, such as access to records from a variety of locations in the NHS, and enable the use of sophisticated information search and retrieval systems. Information and care given can be shared on a 'need to know' basis (Hoy 2009). With the rollout of 'GP2GP', patient records can now be transferred at the touch of a button, rather than patients waiting weeks or months for paper records to be relocated. Patients have the right to opt out from having their record uploaded to the central database and guidance on this is available via the NHS Connecting for Health website.

Concerns have been raised about the security of electronic records, however confidentiality is maintained through strict and robust security measures and access is via smart cards using 'chip and PIN' technology. The level of access is determined by the role of the individual healthcare professional. EPRs offer a number of advantages including ease of access across geographical and organizational boundaries, administration, continuity and accessibility, with all care episodes recorded in one shared record.

Activity

- During your next few shifts in the clinical area, identify how confidentiality is maintained in the clinical environment, with particular reference to the use of technology, such as telephone calls and accessing patient information via the computer.
- Are there any actions you can identify that have the potential to compromise confidentiality in the clinical setting?

Electronic prescribing allows prescribers to send prescriptions electronically to the pharmacy of the patient's choice, making the system safer and more convenient. Such prescribing enhances the security of prescriptions as there are no prescription pads to be lost or stolen and prescriptions cannot be tampered with prior to presentation at the pharmacy. For patients, it means the reduction of travel as they will go directly to the chemist to collect their prescription, and this system may also reduce waiting time at the pharmacy. For the prescriber there will be greater efficiency in the processing of individual prescriptions through the use of electronic signatures. There is the facility to cancel an electronic prescription up to the point when it has been dispensed and to document the reason. There will be no need to sort and post prescriptions, and fees will be claimed electronically, reducing staff time and paper waste.

'Choose and book' is a system that enables patients to select the time, date and location of an initial outpatient appointment in a hospital or clinic. This speeds up the referral process and ensures greater efficiency as the patient can choose without waiting for a letter and allocation of an appointment they may or may not be able to attend. Patients may access this service at their GP surgery, but can also access it from home via the 'Healthspace' website.

Patient perspective

'I take several medicines for my blood pressure. It used to be such a palaver getting my repeat – I had to take a ticked list back to the GP, go back again two days later to pick up my prescription, and then travel to the chemist to have them make up my repeat. Recently I was told I could email the request, and now the doctor sends the prescription electronically to the chemist so I only have to make one journey, which saves me both time and money!'

> **Reflection point**
> Consider the needs of older patients who may not be so familiar with the use of technology or those who may not have access to a computer to request prescriptions and appointments.
>
> - Will all groups be able to work effectively within the technology?
> - Which groups may be disadvantaged by the technology?

Telemedicine

Telemedicine describes the use of technologies that allow the practice of healthcare using telecommunication equipment. IT developments have enabled instant access to specialist knowledge. Traditionally, access to care is provided via GP surgeries, hospital and community teams, and this involves travel, either on the part of the patient or the clinician to engage in a face-to-face consultation. Using new technologies allows the clinician and patient to engage from two separate locations and may allow a clinician access to a highly specialist opinion without the need to travel long distances. Engagement in this area has been utilized and developed extensively by military organizations requiring specialist input out in the field and transfers effectively into civilian circumstances (Tyrell 2002). The technology offers advantages for isolated rural communities and some specialities lend themselves better than others to telemedicine (e.g. dermatology). Development has been ongoing in many specialities including radiology and pathology using sophisticated imaging equipment. Telemedicine can be utilized in both synchronous and asynchronous circumstances, depending on the urgency of the situation. Asynchronous communication is likely to be appropriate in an outpatient scenario, whereas in A&E synchronous communication may be necessary. Many widely available technologies support telemedicine, such as video cameras, video or teleconferencing, mobile telephone devices, the internet and computers themselves. The NHS Direct telephone and internet service is a well-known example of a large, widely used telemedicine project. It comprises a telephone helpline, staffed by trained health professionals, and a website that provides accurate and up-to-date information. It provides remote access to healthcare professionals who are equipped to provide the caller with advice and are able to direct them to the most appropriate service. Other examples include ambulances enabled to transmit data (such as ECG readings) to A&E departments ahead of their arrival to ensure the correct treatment is ready and waiting.

> **Activity**
> Arrange to go and visit a telephone advice service such as NHS Direct.
>
> - Discuss the advantages and limitations of such a service with the staff.
> - Undertake an internet/library search to find studies on the use of telephone services in healthcare.
> - Read these and reflect on them in the light of your experiences.

Telemedicine offers benefits for many areas of healthcare, such as providing patients with remote access to care and enabling clinicians to access specialist advice. It potentially saves time, money and the environmental impact of travel. Disadvantages include the lack of face-to-face interaction and the impact of this upon the clinician–patient relationship. There are ethical and security issues that must be addressed and a need to train staff and adapt working practices to utilize telemedicine, as well as a need to develop contingency plans for equipment failure.

Conclusion

Technology has a vital role to play in the delivery of modern healthcare and in supporting robust and effective communication platforms. This chapter has explored a range of issues relating to the use of IT in healthcare and has encouraged nurses to consider the following issues.

- Developments in technology have changed the ways in which humans interact and communicate in all areas of daily living and now facilitate communication beyond the constraints of fixed time and place.
- Access to healthcare staff and healthcare delivery has been transformed by the integration of IT into the NHS.
- The use of mobile technology needs to be carefully managed by individuals and organizations to avoid potential stress.
- Effective use of the different technologies such as email and mobile phones requires training and quality management to avoid breaches of confidentiality.
- The internet provides a rich source of information to both health professionals and service users. This can support professional development and patient care, but individuals must ensure they verify the quality of the information and validity of its source, ensuring it has a sound evidence base.

References

Bates, D.W. and Gawande, A.A. (2003) Improving safety with information technology, *New England Journal of Medicine*, 348(25): 2526–34.

Bishop, T. (2008) Introducing telephone triage, *Practice Nurse*, 36(4): 43.

Bull, M. (2007) *Sound Moves: iPod Culture and Urban Experience*. London: Routledge.

DH (Department of Health) (2010) *Confidentiality*, www.dh.gov.uk/Publicationsandstatistics/ Publications/PublicationsPolicyAndGuidance/Browsable/DH_5133529 (accessed 28 March 2010).

Gore, P.A. Jr, Leuwerke, W.C. and Krumboltz, J.D. (2002) Technologically enriched and boundaryless lives: time for a paradigm upgrade, *The Counselling Psychologist*, 30(6): 847–57.

Hoy, D. (2009) Going paperless, *Nursing Standard*, 23(25): 23.

Lilley, R.C. (2006) *Dealing with Difficult People*. London: Kogan Page.

NMC (Nursing and Midwifery Council) (2008) *The Code: Standards of Conduct, Performance and Ethics for Nurses and Midwives*, www.nmc-uk.org.uk (accessed 11 March 2010).

Nursing Standard (2009) Misuse of networking sites 'could cost you your job', *Nursing Standard*, 23(26): 10.

Reymond, E. (2008) Facebook: nurses' friend or foe? http://community. healthcarerepublic.com/blogs/editors_blog/archive/2008/11/21/facebook-nurses-friend-or-foe.aspx (accessed 11 March 2010).

Robb, M. (2004) Changing methods of communication, *Nursing Management*, 10(9): 32–5.

Shea, V. (2004) Netiquette, www.albion.com/netiquette/book/index.html (acessed 11 March 2010).

Sully, P. and Dallas, J. (2005) *Essential Communication Skills for Nursing*. Edinburgh: Elservier Mosby.

Tyrell, S. (2002) *Using the Internet in Healthcare*, 2nd edn. Oxford: Radcliffe.

University of Liverpool (2009) Guidelines on the effective use of email, www.liv.ac.uk/csd/email/emailuse.htm (accessed 25 May 2009).

Zittrain, J. (2008) *The Future of the Internet and How to Stop It*. London: Allen Lane.

5 Effective communication in teams

Vivian Jellis

This chapter explores how teams can communicate effectively in healthcare settings. As healthcare professionals we need to acquire effective communication and team-working skills and there are a number of political drivers that have influenced such development. One of the vignettes, concerning a patient named Pearl, is presented to encourage reflection upon how we work in healthcare teams and how we communicate together. Furthermore, this chapter aims to highlight issues concerning the roles of individuals and to consider the issues of leadership and management within teams.

Learning outcomes

By the end of this chapter you should be able to:
1. Understand the difference between leadership and management skills.
2. Appreciate the structure and functions of healthcare teams.
3. Recognize the importance and value of interprofessional communication across teams.

Introduction

Teamwork in healthcare is not a new phenomenon but is fundamental to the delivery of effective, good quality care, to the extent that the concept of teamwork has become embedded within NHS policy. This century has seen a number of policy documents, including *The NHS Plan* (DH 2000), which advocate the need for services to be delivered by teams rather than individual healthcare professionals. Furthermore, *The NHS Plan* states that failure to deliver healthcare priorities is due to a lack of teamwork within the NHS. Teamwork occurs at all levels and policy-makers, managers and those who deliver healthcare services all require skills in team working (Boaden and Leaviss 2000). As the health needs of the population become more complex it is necessary to form healthcare teams with a diverse range of skills to meet the needs of patients. This is highlighted in the long-term conditions

(LTCs) agenda (DH 2005). The vignette in this chapter illustrates the complex nature of patients referred to in this policy. To achieve good quality care for this patient group, collaborative teamwork, in the form of multidisciplinary, interprofessional and integrated working (Fletcher 2008), provides the means by which positive outcomes are achieved. The interface between primary and secondary care will also be examined, as effective communication within and between teams is fundamental to ensuring continuity of care (Hibberd 1998).

Interprofessional teams

Contemporary nursing practice requires healthcare professionals to be equipped with communication and teamworking skills. This is reflected by the professional bodies including the Nursing and Midwifery Council (NMC) and the General Medical Council (GMC), both of which recommend that these areas are integrated into the education of healthcare practitioners (DH 2003). However, one of the major obstacles to interprofessional teamwork is the lack of shared learning between healthcare professionals (Boaden and Leaviss 2000). Nurses, doctors, allied healthcare professionals and social workers are educated independently, which may preclude an understanding of individual professional roles. Teams delivering care to patients with LTCs need to ensure that each role is clarified so that the care delivered is of good quality, appropriate and not duplicated. The development of competency-based education has signalled a move for health and social care workers to develop skills in teamworking. The lack of access to interprofessional learning opportunities is one of the barriers to putting these into practice. Furthermore, as the needs of patients become more complex, the diversity of skills required within the team becomes greater.

Activity

First-time students
- Revisit your practice outcomes and identify the competencies you are expected to achieve relating to communication and teamwork.
- How are you going to achieve these competencies?
- What evidence can you use to support your achievement?

Experienced nurses
- For those of you who are returning to practice or are studying at a higher level, try to reflect on your nurse education and re-examine your competencies in the light of those required by new nursing students.
- Can you remember if teamwork was identified as part of your pre-registration education?
- What differences, if any, do you feel there are between now and then?
- How did you achieve these competencies?

Vignette   End of life care for Pearl

Pearl White is an 85-year-old lady, residing in the community with her husband. Pearl has a history of heart failure, transient ischemic attacks and cerebral
atrophy. Over the past six months she has developed speech and swallowing
difficulties, her dietary intake has reduced, she has lost weight but her BMI is
still over 25. She coughs violently when taking oral fluids and some solids, and
as a result she is reluctant to eat as it is too distressing for her. Pearl's mobility
has also reduced and she has great difficulty moving between her chair and her
bed. Pearl is incontinent of urine and refuses to be catheterized. She has a care
package consisting of four visits per day to maintain personal hygiene, deal with
continence issues, food preparation and feeding.

Pearl was referred by the community matron to the speech and language
therapist and dietician. Video fluoroscopy revealed that Pearl has significant
mechanical swallowing difficulties. She was referred to the gastroenterologist at
the local general hospital and was admitted to hospital for assessment for her
suitability for the insertion of a percutaneous endoscopic gastrostomy (PEG).
Pearl was assessed as having capacity to make her own decisions and following
assessment declined the insertion of the PEG. While in hospital her condition
deteriorated and she became bed-bound, requiring hoisting from bed to chair.
Pearl became very agitated and frightened when hoisted and after discussions
with her and her family she was nursed in bed. Her continence was managed at
this stage with an indwelling catheter.

Pearl and her family were informed of her prognosis as a result of her decision to decline insertion of the PEG. Pearl asked to go home to die. She was
granted continuing healthcare funding and arrangements were made for her to go
home.

The above scenario will be used throughout this chapter to relate some of the
theoretical aspects of teamwork to the everyday practice that nurses undertake in
both primary and secondary care.

Joining a team

Throughout our personal life and professional careers we will join many teams.
Their structure and function will vary, as will our role within the team. There are
numerous definitions of a team (Pritchard and Pritchard 1994). The literature identifies that a team is a divergent group of individuals, who are clear about their role
and the roles of others, who come together and are committed to achieving a common goal. In Pearl's case nurses, doctors, speech and language therapists, dieticians,
occupational therapists, social workers and a discharge planning team were some
of the healthcare professionals involved in delivering care and as such became a
team. The characteristics which made them a team include open communication,

mutual respect for each other, an understanding of their own and their colleagues' roles within the team and a common goal which includes a commitment to provide Pearl with the best quality care. However, none of the above definitions identify the means by which teams form in order to achieve their goals. Moreover, in order for teams to become effective they need to develop a sense of identity and purpose and communicate effectively.

Reflection point
- Think about some of the teams you have been placed with in clinical practice. Identify the teams that you felt were good and those you felt were not so good.
- What characteristics made a good team function well? What was lacking in the not so good team?
- Consider the impact the good team had on delivering patient care compared to the not so good team.

How does an individual join a team? For Pearl, the team was formed as a result of her healthcare needs. The team came together quickly due to the urgency of the situation; there was no time to plan the formation of this team. Successful teamwork doesn't just happen, it takes effort and more than an agreement just to work together (DHSS 1981). Tuckman (1965) described the processes by which teams develop. He identified four stages to the development of an effective team on a continuum from immaturity to maturity:

- *Forming*. Here the members of team are getting to know each other, goals are agreed, but members act independently, rather than as a team. The team caring for Pearl may identify with this as they were in effect 'thrown together'.
- *Storming*. Occurs as the group establishes itself. Team members talk to each other but do not necessarily agree with each other and this can cause conflict. Health-care professionals may associate this with an uncomfortable feeling when joining a new team.
- *Norming*. Here the group sets clear guidelines for practice, begins to work well together and respects each other's contribution to the task. At this stage, members of the team should feel accepted and have a role to play within the team.
- *Performing*. This occurs when the group is working effectively; they trust each other and respect each other's opinions and decisions.

Adjourning was later identified by Tuckman (Tuckman and Jensen 1977) as the fifth stage of team formation. This occurs when a team is disbanded, a common scenario when patients are discharged from hospital to another care setting. This will be evident when Pearl is discharged. The team that came together to meet her care needs will disband and the members may join another team meeting the health needs of other patients. Students should be able to recognize this cycle of events as they progress through their education.

Reflection point
>   Think about a team that you have joined in either your professional career
>   (e.g. a nursing team) or your personal life (e.g. a sports team). Now that
>   you have an understanding of how teams form, try to relate the stages
>   above to one of those teams.

Sully and Dallas (2005) identify the difficulties pre-registration students experience throughout their education. It is difficult to become an effective member of a team when you are continually moving from one placement or team to another in different organizational settings for short periods of time. Effective teamworking may therefore only become a reality when we complete our education and join a substantive team. To overcome this, nurses need effective communication skills, clarity regarding their role and also a clear understanding of their practice outcomes and how they will achieve them within each practice placement. Practical solutions to this problem may include the student actively engaging with the team they are going to join prior to their placement. Making initial introductions, identifying their mentor and ensuring that they are aware of the student's placement dates, learning outcomes and how these outcomes can be achieved need to be discussed at the beginning of the placement. This may help to ensure that when patients like Pearl are admitted some of the initial stages of team development have already been accomplished.

Activity
Reflect on your career to date.

- List the teams that you have joined since commencing your registered nurse education.
- What preparation did you have prior to joining the team?
- How were you introduced to the team?
- How did you feel joining the team?
- At what stage did you feel part of the team and were you able to make a contribution to that team?
- Was there anything you feel could have been done to improve the process of joining the team?

How do teams function?

The main function of any healthcare team is to deliver good quality care. Teams occur at all levels of the NHS from senior management to front-line care delivery. The Harding Committee (DHSS 1981) identified that in order for a team to function effectively it had to have:

- a common objective, accepted and understood by all the members;
- a clear understanding by each team member of their role, function and responsibilities;
- a clear understanding by each team member of the role, function, skills and responsibilities of the other team members;
- a mutual respect for the roles of each team member.

Although this definition is from 1981, it is still relevant to contemporary healthcare today, since all of these characteristics are essential to achieving teamwork in modern healthcare settings and the emphasis on teamworking remains high on the political agenda. However, the definition does not reflect the importance of communication skills as fundamental to team functioning.

As a registered nurse you will be expected to become part of a professional team to deliver good quality healthcare to your client group. The NMC *Code* (NMC 2008: 5) states: 'Work with others to protect and promote the health and wellbeing of those in your care, their families, carers and the wider community'. The *Code* then goes on to specify the prerequisites required to maintain professional teamwork, including cooperation with colleagues, respect for individuals' skills within the team and the sharing of skills, consultation with others within the team and referral to others when appropriate. Teamwork is essential to meet the complex needs of patients like Pearl. Teamwork is not static; it takes energy and motivation to deliver good quality care, hence the team caring for Pearl must act together, their skills must reflect Pearl's complex health needs, they must cooperate to ensure all her needs are met, they must communicate with each other and they must *share* decisions about Pearl's care. At all times throughout the process Pearl should also be acknowledged as part of the team and should be involved in decisions about her care. Xyrichis and Ream (2007) highlight that teamwork will improve outcomes for the patient, the staff and the organization.

One of the major challenges in large organizations such as the NHS is the issue of cross-boundary working. Caring for Pearl requires collaboration between primary and secondary care and Hibberd (1998) identifies three models of such working:

- The first is verbal/written communication, usually in the form of either a letter from the GP advising of reasons for admission/referral and on discharge a letter/fax advising findings and changes to medication. The problem with this form of communication is that as patients' needs become more complex, insufficient details are communicated to the receiving professional. This was certainly the situation for Pearl; the referral only related to the swallowing difficulties and did not include other complex issues.
- The second model is communication through use of a coordinator. Here the multidisciplinary community team and the multidisciplinary hospital team act independently but liaise through a coordinator. The danger with this is that the coordinator is relying on others to pass on information correctly.
- The third model is a 'hospital at home model'. Here, the concept of outreach is central in order to ease the transition from hospital to community and maintain continuity of care. It is suggested that this model reduces organizational

boundaries and enables the smooth transition of care. However, it requires high levels of interaction and communication to facilitate good handover when the outreach is discontinued.

Hibberd also proposes a fourth model, the 'inter-sector teamwork' model. This involves a multidisciplinary team made up of professionals from hospital and community, but which also includes the patient and carers. The group is project-specific: the skills within the team reflect the needs of the patient. This team is transient as it will disband when the goal is achieved and reform in another format to meet the needs of another patient. However, it clearly demonstrates collaboration/communication between healthcare professionals and agencies to provide a 'seamless service' as proposed by *The NHS Plan*.

Activity

- Which team model do you think best reflects Pearl's needs?
- Do you feel the team composition met Pearl's healthcare needs?
- Briefly discuss whether you feel Pearl and her family were part of the team, and if so, why.
- List and describe the role of each member of the team involved in Pearl's care.

Communication within teams

Communication is crucial for the team to function effectively. Effective communication in teams may be hindered by a lack of networking, multiple service providers from different organizations and lack of standardized documentation (the use of electronic patient records – EPRs – is further explored in Chapter 4). Caring for Pearl involved regular meetings with the multidisciplinary team, which included members from primary and secondary care, the review of written goals/outcomes and jointly agreed care packages. Pearl's community matron's perspective is given below.

Team perspective

'As a community matron I could go up to the ward and visit Pearl, but I could also access her medical and nursing records which were all in the same file. I could actively prepare for her discharge and meet with the ward staff face to face. Attending the discharge planning meeting enabled me to meet doctors, nurses, therapists and the discharge planning team so that when Pearl was discharged we had continuity of care. This was really important to me as my role is to coordinate care for Pearl.'

This approach was further facilitated by all healthcare professionals involved in Pearl's care, including community nurses, using a common set of records. Therefore, at any one time any professional involved in Pearl's care could see progress to date.

Accurate record-keeping is fundamental to good communication, however Peters *et al.* (1996) identify that despite overwhelming research evidence, record-keeping continues to be poor in quality and not fit for purpose. Changes are in progress with the introduction of Connecting for Health (see Chapter 4) and EPRs, which all healthcare professionals will be able to access.

Vignette   Delayed care

Lucia is a 75-year-old lady with bilateral leg ulcers which have not responded to treatment. She has been referred to the tissue viability nurse for reassessment. Following assessment the nurse prescribes a new dressing regime and makes a record in Lucia's notes. At the next visit the community staff nurse reads the notes but is not able to implement the changes as the dressings have not been requested. As a result Lucia's care is delayed.

Activity

What issues may have hindered effective communication in the above situation? Suggest how these issues may be addressed.

Giving and receiving feedback

When working as part of a team, giving and receiving feedback is a fundamental skill. Feedback should be used as a tool to help other people or team members to develop or change in a way that improves their behaviour, thinking or skills. Thus the first step is to seek permission to give feedback. Health professionals may tend to focus on negative situations, and while it is good to be able to analyse a situation when things have not gone well, it is equally important to recognize when things have gone particularly well, so that they can be built upon. It is also important that there is time and space to concentrate on feedback.

The aim of feedback is to be constructively critical and supportive while being honest. It is 'not just to provide a judgement and evaluation. It is to provide insight. Without insight into their own strengths and limitations [trainees] cannot progress to resolve difficulties' (King 1999: 2). There are various 'rules and guidelines' on how to give feedback. It is paramount to ensure that the receiver is at the centre of whatever process is chosen and that the feedback is balanced. The process below is derived from various sources (King 1999; Pendleton *et al.* 2003; Silverman *et al.* 2005).

Vignette   Marut's first dressing

Marut, a first-year student nurse, has just successfully changed his first dressing on a restless patient. His mentor, Kazia, would like to give him some positive feedback. She approaches him and asks: 'Marut, I was wondering if you have

10 minutes so that I could talk to you about how you thought that dressing went?' Marut feels a little worried and says he thought he probably did some things wrong and starts to list all the negative aspects. Kazia allows him to continue, resisting the temptation to rescue him immediately, but instead, as he articulates his thoughts, she encourages him to suggest solutions to the issues he raises and adds her own suggestions as well. Kazia particularly makes a point of raising the aspects that had gone well, and summarizes both the achievements and the points for improvement.

Team member roles and attributes

The recent explosion of new roles in healthcare (Read/ENRip team 1999) will impact upon the cohesiveness and effectiveness of the team, especially if there is a lack of clarity about a person's role within that team. In order for a team to be effective, members must be clear about their own roles and those of the rest of the team (Belbin 2002). Furthermore, the actual composition of the team is crucial to achieving the desired outcomes.

Belbin (2002: 22) found that in order for a team to be effective, certain roles have to be adopted by the team members. Belbin identifies the following nine roles within a team, with their corresponding attributes:

- *Plant.* Creative, imaginative, unorthodox, but with the ability to solve difficult problems.
- *Resource investigator.* Extrovert, enthusiastic, communicative, exploring all opportunities and developing contacts.
- *Coordinator.* Mature, confident, a good chairperson. Clarifies goals, promotes decision-making, delegates well.
- *Shaper.* Challenging, dynamic, thrives on pressure. Has the drive and courage to overcome obstacles.
- *Monitor evaluator.* Sober, strategic and discerning. Has the ability to see all options. A good judge.
- *Team worker.* Cooperative, mild, perceptive and diplomatic. Listens, builds, averts friction and calms the waters.
- *Implementer.* Disciplined, reliable, conservative and efficient. Good at turning ideas into practical actions.
- *Completer/finisher.* Painstakingly conscientious, gets very anxious at times. Searches out errors and omissions, but always delivers on time.
- *Specialist.* Single minded, self-starting, dedicated. Provides knowledge and skills to the team in rare supply.

Belbin proposes that each of the above team roles is required in order for a team to be effective, and he also differentiates between 'team role' and 'functional role', which is very evident in healthcare. We all have a functional role, be it nurse, doctor, therapist etc., but *team roles* are more to do with how you conduct yourself, contribute and relate to the other members of the team. Therefore, in caring for Pearl, we would have two roles, our functional role and our team role.

Effective teams need good management and leadership (Hayes 2002). The skills required to manage a team are different to those required to lead one, but they are not mutually exclusive – in fact, Contino (2004) contends that management and leadership skills are very similar. The team manager has overarching responsibility for the team and is responsible for ensuring the organizational goals/objectives are achieved. The manager achieves this through facilitation of the team, ensuring that the resources required are available to the team, that the skill mix within the team is appropriate to the task and that they give as much support to the team as needed (Martin 2000a). Managers also need to ensure that their teams communicate effectively; if a manager has poor communication skills then this may be reflected in the team's ability to communicate effectively. Managers can facilitate good communication with their teams by actively seeking feedback about their own communication skills and also by ensuring that their staff have the knowledge and skills to communicate effectively. This may involve sending staff to workshops/training for communication skills.

Within the NHS two scenarios exist: some clinicians become managers, but many managers are not clinicians and enter the NHS through graduate management schemes, which may impact on the way the team is managed, especially a clinical team. As a result, managers may be described as functioning *outside* the team, whereas team leaders are seen as functioning *within* the team. Martin (2000b) contends that if you use the term 'team leader' it implies that only one person can be the team leader, however if you use the term 'team leadership' it implies a position that can be fulfilled by anyone depending on the skills of the individual and the task at hand. The introduction of 'clinical leaders', whose main role is the development of clinical practice (with no management role), has also been seen as a means of developing communication skills and has been achieved by the clinical lead taking responsibility for clinical supervision, mentorship and maintaining clinical records.

- *Leadership* skills include, organizational management, communication, analysing/strategy and the ability to create a vision (Contino 2004).
- *Organizational* management includes managing time, people and resources.
- *Communication* skills include exchanging information, talking, listening, being challenged in a non-threatening environment, motivating staff.
- *Strategy* skills include shared decision-making, knowledge of the team's outcomes/business plans and vision, creating opportunities for the team, including the opportunity to lead, and ensuring continuous professional development (CPD) for the team.

Activity

Think about your current placement and list the roles undertaken by the staff.

- Who is the leader?
- Who is the manager?

Belbin suggests that we can adopt different roles.

- Which of Belbin's team roles do you feel describes you in your current placement?
- Which of these roles most suits you, and why?
- Identify the positive attributes within the team. Are there any qualities that the team needs to develop?

Working in teams

Various teams exist within primary and secondary care and their structure and function is dependent upon a number of elements, including the organizational structure, the client group and the care setting. A number of team structures can be identified within healthcare including multiprofessional teams, multidisciplinary teams and interprofessional teams. Scholes and Vaughan (2002) clarify the difference between these teams, highlighting that the multiprofessional team comes from different health and social care backgrounds, but may not act together. The primary healthcare team is a good example of this. The multidisciplinary team has members who share the same professional background but practise within different specialities or branches – for example, district nurse, respiratory specialist nurse, intensive care nurse. Finally, 'interprofessional' refers to interactions between team members. Scholes and Vaughan also highlight that within government policy these terms are used interchangeably. Team working is the means by which teams interact in order to achieve their common goal. In order to be effective, teams need to be developed. They not only need a common goal to work towards but also require a clear function, need to be organized, to have good communication strategies and policies and guidelines in place. Due to the increasingly complex healthcare needs of patients, teams are expanding to include a range of healthcare professionals and as such will need to recognize the contribution of each team member in order to remain effective.

Reflection point
Think about the team you are currently placed with.

- What healthcare professionals make up your team?
- Can you identify who belongs to the multidisciplinary team and who belongs to the multiprofessional team?

Senior management teams may have no direct contact with patients but will be required to provide the resources to deliver services to those patients (Boaden and Leaviss 2000). These may be described as 'indirect teams' because of the lack of front-line patient contact, whereas teams delivering patient care are seen as 'direct teams'. In contemporary healthcare there are a variety of different teams, including 'project teams', which may be set up to improve the quality of a service or to develop a new service. 'Care delivery teams' may be further divided into client-specific groups such as children, care of the elderly or learning disability teams. 'Disease-specific teams' include respiratory, cardiac, stroke and neurological disease teams (CHSRF 2006). These teams may be multiprofessional – that is, composed of professionals from different health and social care backgrounds – or 'uniprofessional', as in specialist nurse teams. In addition, teams are recognized on the basis of where care is delivered, such as primary care, secondary care and long-term care.

Øvretveit (1993) identifies three further types of team:

- *The client team* is formed by a group of professionals from different backgrounds who come together specifically to provide care for an individual patient. They may not meet face to face but do communicate. This team is transient and disbands when the care episode has ended or the patient's needs have changed.
- *The network association team* comprises volunteers who act as a vessel for making referrals to other professionals.
- *Formal teams* are multidisciplinary and are governed by policy, with an identified team leader – for example, the primary healthcare team.

Pre-registration students will become part of a number of teams and will need to recognize that the nature of the team will reflect the task/goal they are required to achieve. The composition of the team will vary depending on the task/goal. The more complex the task, the more complex the group. In the case of Pearl, the team caring for her is best reflected in the client team: the team did meet, but disbanded when Pearl was discharged.

Vignette	**Pearl's discharge planning meeting**
Nurse:	If I may start, Pearl has now been on the ward for a week. She has been assessed under the Mental Capacity Act and has capacity to make her own decisions. She has refused the insertion of a PEG and understands the consequences of this decision. She would like to go home to die.
Doctor:	I agree with Pearl's decision. The procedure would have been very difficult and the risks are high, as Pearl has complex health problems. As long as Pearl and her family are aware that she is going home for end of life care, then we can plan for her discharge as soon as possible.
Community matron:	I'm happy for Pearl to be discharged, but I do have concerns about how Mr White will manage as he has his own health problems. He's deaf and sleeps upstairs. He won't hear Pearl if she's choking.
Social worker:	We can arrange a package of care. I have fast-tracked continuing healthcare under the palliative care criteria and the package will be in place by the end of the week. This will include a night sit.

Dietician:	I'm happy for Pearl to go home, but I will need time to prepare the family and carers to ensure Pearl's dietary needs are met. I have discussed this with the speech and language therapist and we have agreed a consistency of food appropriate to Pearl's needs.
Occupational therapist:	I'll contact the family to undertake a home visit. I need to assess access for a profiling bed and mattress. Pearl refuses to be hoisted so carers must use sliding sheets to move Pearl. I'll prepare a manual handling plan.
Social worker:	I'll contact the care agency and hospital at home to ensure that they are aware of Pearl's care plan.
Doctor:	As everyone is in agreement that Pearl should go home, we can start discharge planning today.

The discharge planning meeting outlined above epitomizes good teamwork among healthcare professionals. However, one aspect in which it is lacking is that the patient and/or their representative were not present at the meeting and so were unable to offer their perspective. However, it did demonstrate that there was no hierarchy among the healthcare professionals; there is evidence of open communication and shared decision-making, questions are asked and all avenues are explored in order to facilitate a successful discharge.

Patient perspective

Later, Mr White commented: 'I am sorry I could not attend your meeting but it is nice that the staff have asked our views about Pearl coming home and how I would manage. I know Pearl wants to come home, but at my age I need to be considered as well.'

Activity

- Access a discharge planning meeting in as many of your clinical placements as possible.
- Reflect on the meeting and try to identify which healthcare professional played which of Belbin's team roles. For example, who would you say was the 'plant' and why?
- What elements can you identify that would lead you to believe that this was a good example of an effective team?
- How did the team members demonstrate that they had a good understanding of their own role and those of the rest of the team?
- Do you feel that the team showed mutual respect, and if so how?

Hierarchies

As a student nurse you may have experienced or identified hierarchies within your clinical placements. The discharge planning meeting described above demonstrates a 'flattened' team structure which acknowledges the roles and responsibilities of each of the members of the team. *The NHS Plan* advocates that teamworking should replace the old hierarchies which exist within the NHS and that hierarchical structures should be replaced with good leadership (Xyrichis and Ream 2007). Hierarchy has been blamed for failure in teamwork and team working has been identified as a means of replacing hierarchy (Martin 2000b). Effective teams usually contain a combination of experience and expertise and rarely have a hierarchy. However, Martin (2000b) suggests that there are situations when a hierarchical leadership style is evident and this occurs when the team leader also has managerial responsibility. In this situation the leader expects the team to follow and does not attempt to empower the team. Without the team being empowered, power will remain seated with the team leader and not with the team. If the team is not empowered it will not function effectively.

The team caring for Pearl may be seen as an empowered team, taking a democratic approach to communication. They met face to face, all their views were taken into consideration, the team contributed to the discussions about Pearl's care and became involved in problem-solving, culminating in shared decision-making. There was a consensus of opinion that Pearl should go home to die, there was discussion about the care needs identified and each healthcare professional identified their role within the discharge plan. Furthermore, there was acknowledgement of the family's needs and Pearl's right to make her own decisions and be involved in her care.

In a hierarchical team, the team leader traditionally would have been the consultant and would have led the meeting. It would have been their clinical decision as to whether or not Pearl was discharged and there would have been little or no shared decision-making. The consultant would have given instructions as to what he thought Pearl's needs were and allocated tasks to individuals as they thought best. Communication would have been 'top down', and would not have allowed other healthcare professionals to give their views or opinions.

Reflection point

As a student you should be able to recognize your own feelings of being empowered or led.

- Think about whether your current role as a student enables you to be empowered or do you feel you are always led?

Tribalism

As the healthcare needs of patients become more complex and the numbers of healthcare professionals involved in caring for patients with LTCs increases, there is a danger that *tribalism* will occur. Tribalism is defined as 'the state of existing as a separate tribe' and has been identified as a major obstacle to integrated and collective working within the NHS (Van Der Weyden 2006). Tribalism is not unique to the medical profession but also extends throughout nursing and other healthcare professions and can impact upon communication within and between teams.

Since the inception of the NHS there has been a gradual erosion of professional boundaries. Many healthcare professionals have seen their roles develop to encompass new skills and knowledge, many of which were traditionally seen as the remit of the doctor. For example, in the case of Pearl, the community matron made the initial referral to both the speech and language therapist and the dietician, whereas previously only a doctor would have made such referrals. This reflects the expansion of new roles which has been influenced by the reduction of junior doctors' working hours (DH 2001), changing patterns of medical education and changing models of care.

Recent government policy dictates that our current workforce must be more flexible in their professional roles: 'Our objective is to liberate the talents and skills of all the workforce so that every patient gets the right care in the right place at the right time' (DH 2002: 34). Traditional roles in healthcare are changing, professional boundaries are being pushed and nurses are taking on roles which were traditionally the remit of doctors, including non-medical prescribing for community matrons and in the case of Pearl and the speech and language therapist, the ability to request video fluoroscopy. In 1999, the Department of Health commissioned a study entitled *Exploring New Roles In Practice* (ENRip) (Read/ENRip team 1999). This study identified that in the 40 acute NHS Trusts studied, there were 838 new roles, 72 per cent carried out by nurses and 28 per cent by allied health professionals. This has significant implications for healthcare professionals as such an expansion of responsibilities demands greater communication skills in order to ensure that everyone is aware of individual roles and responsibilities.

Vignette   'Not my job'

Raj is the only staff nurse on the ward. He is not competent to insert intravenous cannulae. He calls the house officer to re-canulate Mrs Smith as her intravenous infusion has tissued and she is due her intravenous drugs. The house officer says this is not his job, and Raj should get the physician's assistant to do it.

Reflection point

Consider the scenario above. Have you ever experienced an 'it's not my job' situation? If so, what was the impact on you and your patient?

Several examples of initiatives to overcome tribalism have been published. Kinley *et al.* (2001) undertook a randomized control trial examining the skills of highly trained nurses versus those of house officers in the assessment of preoperative surgical day patients. The study concluded that there is capacity for flexibility in professional roles and traditional boundaries should not be allowed to impede patient care. The development of a preoperative assessment tool used by nurses and developed collaboratively with anaesthetists has gone some way to breaking down barriers and has resulted in better communication, reduced tribalism and greater cooperation.

One new role that has challenged traditional norms and benefited the role of nurses in many settings has been the introduction of non-medical prescribing (NMP). This has been one of the most controversial role changes this century and while many doctors are very supportive of NMP, it has not been universally welcomed. In the 'old days', doctors prescribed, pharmacists dispensed and nurses administered medications. Nurses, pharmacists and other professions who have undertaken further training can now prescribe prescription-only medicines, traditionally the domain of medical practitioners only. This has improved patient care by providing better and quicker access to medicines, but it has also increased the need for good communication between doctors and non-medical prescribers. For example, if the community matron prescribes for Pearl she must ensure that this is entered onto the GP's database, as failure to do so could result in the GP or another non-medical prescriber prescribing without up-to-date information.

Waters (1999) contends that as a result of nurses taking on increased responsibility, tribalism will increase rather than diminish. Multiprofessional education has been identified as a means by which tribalism can be overcome. Seabrook (1998) describes a programme of multiprofessional education comprising teamwork and communication skills. Delivered by nurses to first-year medical students, one of the intended outcomes was to facilitate the erosion of barriers between nurses and doctors.

Vignette   'Maxi-nurses'

Naresh is a community matron. She has advanced clinical skills and is an NMP. It is 4 p.m. on a Friday afternoon and she visits Vera, her last visit of the day. Vera has chronic obstructive pulmonary disease (COPD), hypertension and type 2 diabetes. Vera complains that she feels unwell, she is pyrexial, has increased cough, breathlessness and green sputum. Naresh diagnoses Vera with an infective exacerbation of her COPD and prescribes Amoxicillin 500 mgs TDS for seven days and Prednisilone 30 mgs daily for five days. The prescription is given to Vera's husband for immediate collection.

Patient perspective

Vera's husband said of the above: 'The fact that Naresh can prescribe means that we do not have to wait for an appointment after the weekend, nor do we have to call a GP out over the weekend, Vera can get started on her tablets straight away.'

Activity

- Discuss with your mentor/colleague how nurses' roles have changed, and how this relates to communication skills.
- Consider the scenario above. How has the introduction of NMP benefitted patients like Vera?
- Identify some roles which were initially carried out by other healthcare professionals and are now undertaken by nurses.
- How has the change in nurse roles impacted on the team?
- How can health professionals overcome tribalism to improve patient care?

Conclusion

Teamwork is essential for the delivery of effective, good quality healthcare, especially as the needs of the population become more complex. Fundamental to teamwork is good communication. We need to be able to work and communicate effectively as members of a number of teams. The following points have been discussed:

- Healthcare professionals need to understand how to join a team and their role within the team in order to communicate effectively.
- Effective strategies for improving communication between and within multi-professional teams need to be developed. These include face-to-face meetings, good record-keeping, report writing and improved information technology (IT) skills.
- Although management and leadership skills have some similarities, the way in which managers and clinical leaders utilize these skills varies, but both demand high levels of communicative ability.
- Barriers such as hierarchies and tribalism within teams can be overcome with good communication and interprofessional education.

References

Belbin, R.M. (2002) *Team Roles at Work*. Oxford: Butterworth Heinemann.

Boaden, N. and Leaviss, J. (2000) Putting teamwork in context, *Medical Education*, 34: 921–7.

CHSRF (Canadian Health Services Research Foundation) (2006) *Teamwork in Healthcare: Promoting Effective Teamwork in Healthcare in Canada*, www.fcrss.ca (accessed 17 January 2009).

Contino, D. (2004) Leadership competencies: knowledge, skills and aptitudes nurses need to lead organisations effectively, *Critical Care Nurse*, 24(3): 52–64.

DH (Department of Health) (2000) *The NHS Plan*. London: The Stationery Office.

DH (Department of Health) (2001) *Investment and Reform for NHS Staff – Taking Forward the NHS Plan*. London: The Stationery Office.

DH (Department of Health) (2002) *Delivering the NHS Plan*. London: The Stationery Office.

DH (Department of Health) (2003) *Learning for Collaborative Practice with Other Professional Agencies.* London: The Stationery Office.

DH (Department of Health) (2005) *Supporting People with Long Term Conditions. An NHS and Social Care Model to Support Local Innovation and Integration.* London: The Stationery Office.

DHSS (Department of Health and Social Security) (1981) *The Primary Healthcare Team. The Harding Report of a Joint Working Group of the Standing Medical Advisory Committee and the Standard Nursing and Midwifery Committee.* London: DHSS.

Fletcher, M. (2008) Multi-disciplinary teamworking: building and using the team, *Practice Nurse,* 35(12): 42–7.

Hayes, N. (2002) *Managing Teams: A Strategy for Success.* Australia: Thompson Learning.

Hibberd, P.A. (1998) The primary/secondary interface. Cross boundary teamwork – missing link for seamless care? *Journal of Clinical Nursing,* 7(3): 274–82.

King, J. (1999) Giving feedback, *British Medical Journal,* 318(7200): 2.

Kinley, H. Czoski-Murray, C., George, S. *et al.* (2001) Extended scope of nursing practice: a multicentre randomised controlled trial of appropriately trained nurse and pre-registration house officers in pre-operative assessment in elective general surgery, *Health Technology Assessment,* 5(20): 1–87.

Martin, V. (2000a) Developing team effectiveness, *Nursing Standard,* 7(2): 26–9.

Martin, V. (2000b) Effective team leadership, *Nursing Standard,* 7(3): 26–9.

NMC (Nursing and Midwifery Council) (2008) *The Code: Standards of Conduct, Performance and Ethics for Nurses and Midwives,* www.nmc-uk.org.uk (accessed 11 March 2010).

Øvretveit, J. (1993) *Co-ordinating Community Care: Multi-disciplinary Teams and Care Management.* Buckingham. Open University Press.

Pendleton, D.T., Schofield, T., Tate, P. and Havelock, P. (2003) *The New Consultation: Developing Doctor Patient Communication.* Oxford: Oxford University Press.

Peters, A.L., Legorreta, A.P., Ossorio, R.C. and Davidson, M.B. (1996) Quality of outpatient care provided to patients: a health maintenance organisation experience, *Diabetic Care,* 19(6): 601–6.

Pritchard, P. and Pritchard, J. (1994) *Teamwork for Primary and Shared Care.* Oxford: Oxford University Press.

Read, S./ENRip team (1999) *Exploring New Roles in Practice: Implications of Developments Within the Clinical Team (ENRiP). Executive Summary.* Sheffield: School of Health Related Research (ScHARR), University of Sheffield.

Scholes, J. and Vaughan, B. (2002) Cross-boundary working: implications for the multi-professional team, *Journal of Clinical Nursing,* 11(3): 399–408.

Seabrook, M. (1998) Overcoming tribalism, *Nursing Standard,* 12(20): 23–4.

Silverman, J.S., Kurtz, S. and Draper, J. (2005) *Skills for Communicating with Patients.* Oxford: Radcliffe Medical Press.

Sully, P. and Dallas, J. (2005) *Essential Communication Skills for Nursing.* Edinburgh: Elsevier Mosby.

Tuckman, B. (1965) Developmental sequence in small groups, *Psychology Bulletin,* 63: 384–9.

Tuckman, B. and Jensen, M. (1977) Stages of small group development revisited, *Group Organisational Studies,* 2: 419–27.

Van Der Weyden, M. (2006) Leadership and medical tribalism, *Medical Journal of Australia,* 185(7): 345.

Waters, A. (1999) Professional tribalism will increase as nurses accept greater responsibility, *Nursing Standard,* 13(36): 5.

Xyrichis, A. and Ream, E. (2007) Teamwork: a concept analysis, *Journal of Advanced Nursing,* 61(2): 232–41.

6 Communicating with diverse groups

Jill Toocaram

This chapter explores barriers to communication and consulting with disadvantaged and vulnerable groups of people, including people with learning disabilities, physical disabilities, sensory deprivation and cross-cultural issues. Prejudice and stereotyping are common barriers that affect communication and consultation by the devaluing of others within society. This chapter is aimed primarily at helping adult nurses and other professionals understand enough about working with vulnerable groups in order to work more confidently with people as individuals in mainstream settings.

Learning outcomes

By the end of this chapter you should be able to:
1 Demonstrate knowledge and understanding of the difficulties encountered by diverse groups of patients in engaging with healthcare professionals and with particular emphasis on the care of people with learning disabilities.
2 Develop awareness of specific communication skills that will facilitate consulting with diverse groups of patients.

Introduction

Stereotyping people who are different from us often exposes them to oppression and discrimination which exclude such people from mainstream life (e.g. inaccessible buildings or information). Thomas (1999) referred to two types of barrier. There are 'barriers to doing' which restrict what people can do; for example, steps into buildings with no wheelchair access or lifts, written leaflets which cannot be read because people are blind, speak a different language, or have a learning difficulty or disability. There are 'barriers to being' caused by the hurtful or hostile attitudes and/or behaviour of other people, restricting those discriminated against to what they can 'be' or 'become' by damaging their self-esteem and confidence. According to Prothero *et al.* (2009), healthcare professionals are still working in systems that exclude or disadvantage large numbers of people needing care because of sexism, racism, ageism and the inequitable distribution of resources.

Vignette   Power and prejudice

Rosie is a 32-year-old woman who has Down's syndrome and lives at home with her 70-year-old mother. Rosie has severe learning disabilities but is generally quite a happy and content individual. However, over the past year Rosie's behaviour has become more challenging and she has started to self-harm by banging the sides of her face with her hand. She has also had screaming and swearing episodes. Following a full nursing assessment and GP referral, it was confirmed that Rosie had developed cataracts which required treatment. She was seen on four separate occasions over a two-year period by a consultant who finally confirmed he did not feel Rosie was a suitable candidate because she had Down's syndrome with behavioural problems and could not read anyway.

Activity

- Do you agree with the consultant's decision in the above vignette?
- How do you think Rosie's mother feels?
- Write down the barriers you think Rosie is experiencing.
- Reflect on the impact of medical power and authority on Rosie.

What is learning disability?

Learning disability is a generic term which includes people who do not reach their full potential because of arrested, incomplete or interrupted development of the brain, as a result of the impact of 'something' that occurred before, during or after birth. That 'something' covers a very broad area of possibilities and the causes often bring with them significant associated health problems. According to *Signposts for Success* (DH 1998), learning disability is a term used in the UK to describe 'people who have a significant impairment of intelligence and social functioning acquired before adulthood. Educational services in the UK use the term learning difficulty and only those children with moderate or severe learning difficulty would usually be regarded as having a learning disability'. It is worth noting at this point that for most people having a learning *disability* is not the same as having a learning *difficulty*. A learning difficulty is something anyone can have, whether they have a learning disability or not. For instance, a person might have a learning difficulty with sums, academic writing style or how to preset the video recorder, but with help and education these difficulties can be overcome. Many people are increasingly being diagnosed with dyslexia (including student nurses), which is a learning difficulty rather than a learning disability and was misdiagnosed, or not diagnosed at all, in previous years. Dyslexia is a learning difficulty that causes problems with learning language-based skills. It is a neurological condition that affects 10–20 per cent of the population to some degree. However, dyslexia has no effect on your intelligence; it is about *access* to intelligence (Dore 2010).

Healthcare and people with a learning disability

Having a learning disability does not mean a person can never learn something new, but generally speaking that person can never fully overcome the disability. However, given time and patience, many people can be successful at some things despite their disability. An independent inquiry into access to healthcare for people with learning disabilities, conducted in 2008 by Sir Jonathan Mitchell and launched in response to Mencap's report *Death by Indifference* (2007), revealed some examples of good practice, but also examples of discrimination, abuse and neglect across the range of health services. The report makes very sober reading and highlights something written by a learning disability nurse that everybody should remember: 'People with learning disabilities are a touchstone for standards of civilisation in our society. If they are accorded the value and dignity and equality to which they are entitled, then all of us are safer in our rights' (Brooke 1999).

A disability is not an illness and cannot be cured, but people with disabilities are likely to experience a much greater range and intensity of health problems than the rest of the population and also to experience barriers in accessing healthcare. Disorders and many syndromes with associated disabilities, such as physical and sensory disabilities, carry unique health risks and may pose barriers to communication, which carers and health staff must be aware of.

People with learning and other disabilities can have a range of communication difficulties: epilepsy, sensory impairments, behavioural phenotypes and physical disorders including pain, psychological stress and mental health problems (DH 1998). Approximately 15–30 per cent of people with learning disabilities have epilepsy, presenting greater diagnostic problems due to communication issues and in terms of cooperating with the investigations required (DH 1998).

For most people with learning disabilities, the impact of communication difficulties can be minimized with patience and consistent implementation of various interventions and strategies over time. For some individuals the impact will be minor. For others the impact will be significant in terms of their quality of life, and life opportunities, independence, education, health, work, sexuality, relationships and parenting. For a significant minority the impact will be severe.

The Disability Rights Commission investigation (DRC 2006), *Equal Treatment: Closing the Gap*, reviewed 8 million primary care records of people with mental illness and learning disabilities and found they are more likely to die younger and less likely to receive appropriate treatment, investigations and screening. Mencap (2007) investigated the deaths of six people with a learning disability who had died in hospital and concluded that these deaths were preventable and had occurred as a result of poor medical practice. Mencap also concluded that institutional discrimination was widespread within the NHS and that the needs of one of the most vulnerable, stigmatized and excluded groups of people were not being fulfilled.

To summarize, there is a large and varied spectrum of individuals whose lives are affected by the impact of their disability. There is no 'one size fits all' approach.

Autism

Autism is a general term that is used interchangeably with 'pervasive developmental disorders' (PDDs). Individuals with a PDD have a unique set of symptoms that affect communication, socialization (interaction with others) and behaviour. For more information on autism please visit www.exploringautism.org, the site sponsored by National Alliance for Autism Research.

Sometimes people with autism may have a significant learning disability but look completely normal. A person with autism may have limited communication skills and may not talk to or seek to interact with others. Other people can quickly become alarmed and feel quite threatened, and this can impact on effective communication, however, most people tend to be very understanding once they know someone has autism, but it is difficult to balance the giving of personal information while maintaining the privacy and dignity of the individual concerned at the same time. Equally, people without obvious disability would not like or agree to their personal information being constantly broadcast to everyone they meet. Consider the next vignette.

Vignette   Understanding differences and the unexpected

Syed is a 29-year-old Asian man with an autistic spectrum disorder (ASD), who was admitted to the ward with appendicitis. The nurse was helping Syed out of bed to use the commode when from beyond the curtain came the noise of the floor-polishing machine. Syed screamed, pushed the nurse, tipped over the commode and hid under the bed. The nurse was shocked and Syed would not stop screaming. The ward sister appeared and asked the nurse what was going on. The nurse replied that as she was assisting Syed out of bed, he began screaming for no reason and pushed her away. In the process, he knocked over the commode and hid under the bed.

Activity

- What might be the reasons for Syed behaving the way he did?
- Identify what to do next and how.
- Who can help you manage this situation well?
- What would have prevented this incident happening?
- Syed is Asian – does this make him different and would you treat him differently?

Reflection point

- Think about how nurses can be helped to understand the needs of their individual patients.
- How would you prepare yourself to cope better with a similar situation in the future?

Patient perspective

'If I could talk I would tell you something like: "I'm very frightened; there are strange smells, sounds and people. Someone is touching me – aggggh – What's that monster behind the curtain – HELP! HELP! HELP! Don't touch me, don't touch me, and don't touch me. I HURT."'

Communicating with people with learning disabilities

Every conscious person can communicate regardless of the severity of their disability. If nurses can embrace and practice a total communication approach with vulnerable groups of people including the elderly, children, people with mental health problems, people with learning disabilities, the physically disabled and people with sensory deficits, then they should be able to communicate well with everyone else. While not necessarily vulnerable, it is also important to consider the needs of people from other cultures and minority groups.

Reflection point
- Identify what communication approaches you use on a daily basis.
- Do you use different communication methods for friends, family and patients or do you use the same?
- Reflect on your own personal communication philosophy.

Activity

How do you rate your own communication skills out of a score of 1–10?

a) 1–4
b) 5–7
c) 8–10

(1–4 very poor, poor, weak, challenged; 5–7 fair, not bad, average; 8–10 good, very good, excellent)

- If you chose (a) or (b), identify how you can improve your skills.
- If you chose (c), identify why you think you are a good communicator.
- Whatever you have chosen, ask your colleagues if they agree with you.

With changes in neonatal care and increased use of medical technologies – for example, assisted ventilation – more children with complex needs are surviving into adulthood, requiring a high level of skilled care. For example, dementia occurs at a much higher rate among elderly people with learning disabilities than among the general population, which is independent of the association between dementia and Down's syndrome (Cooper 1997). Pain management is particularly important for people who do not easily communicate their discomfort. Confusing displays of challenging behaviour may be difficult to interpret, even for the most experienced carer or professional. Sensitive and well developed observation and communication skills are essential to ascertain the cause (such as a behavioural phenotype, stress, pain or other emotional or physical turmoil). There may be simple solutions such as needing the toilet, a drink, a favourite toy, feeling too hot or cold, or anxiety regarding a new person; or more complex interventions may be required. By working with carers, family and friends, the nurse can ensure that such needs, whether simple or more significant (such as severe pain), are communicated, understood and the appropriate care given. Just because a person has difficulty communicating does not mean they do not have all the same range of emotions and feelings as any other human being.

Poor communication may exert a negative effect on the way people behave. This is particularly noticeable with people who have a learning disability and the way they behave and express themselves. The basic principles of communication with people who have a learning disability are the same as those applied to everyone else: they must be treated with dignity, care and respect (see Chapter 3). However, this is easier said than done if you do not have the communication skills, knowledge and awareness to do so. Firstly, nurses need to develop good verbal skills, speaking clearly and slowly and using simple language. A common error is to rush people before they have had a chance to digest what you are saying to them and not allowing them time to answer. Good listening skills require much patience and must not be underestimated. These skills will develop over time. Alongside listening it is crucial to use observation skills as sometimes people may answer in one way verbally but their body language may be telling you something different. Generally, people like to please others by telling them what they think they would like to hear, and this is often experienced when a person responds with 'Yes' they are 'OK' when in fact they are not. How often have you seen a clinically unwell patient respond when you ask them how they are feeling with, 'I'm fine thank you.' Any nurse who walks away at this point needs to consider their communication skills.

Sign language

Nurses can sometimes overestimate a person's understanding of, or ability to access, verbal language or may fail to identify non-verbal behaviour as a means of communication. Not everyone with a learning disability can talk or hear and they may be using sign language to communicate. There are different types of sign language and resources to aid communication, some more formal than others, for example, British Sign Language (BSL) and the Paget Gorman sign system. These languages vary in how the signs are made with hand shape and position and also how many grammatical markers such as tense and plurality they convey. The Makaton Vocabulary Development Project used signs from BSL to develop a vocabulary of signs which are relevant to the experience and needs of people with learning disabilities. 'Signalong' works on similar principles. Some people with severe disabilities may be able to point to symbols and pictures to explain how they are feeling or what they want or need. Good eye contact and 'eye pointing' become meaningful and communicative and can speak volumes.

Service provision

Services must be responsive to individuals' needs and choices, and patients should be able to match their healthcare needs with their personal preferences. However, for meaningful choice to become a reality there must be a rebalancing of the relationship between users and service providers. Patient choice will only benefit those who can express their preferences and nurses on the front line have it in their power to ensure that this includes people with communication difficulties. The Nursing and Midwifery Council's *Code* (NMC 2008) states: 'make the care of people your first concern, treating them as individuals and respecting their dignity' and 'work with others to protect and promote the health and wellbeing of those in your care, their families and the wider community'. This includes all people with or without disabilities, regardless of sex, race or religion.

Reflection point

People with learning disabilities experience barriers in accessing healthcare.

- Think about how you might explain a procedure, such as a cervical screening test, breast screening or other procedure to a woman who does not have a learning disability compared to a woman with a learning disability, such as Down's syndrome.

Further information, advice and resources can be found by accessing the Cancer Screening website www.cancerscreening.nhs.uk and looking at the leaflets designed for people with a learning disability. The Department of Health (DH) has leaflets on consent that are designed to be accessible to people with learning disabilities.

This chapter now moves on to consider the impact and needs of those with physical disabilities and the impact of other potential barriers with regard to communication skills.

Cultural influences

Cultural and religious practices can vary widely and have a significant impact on communication. In some cultures, those who have a disability may be referred to as being 'gifted', 'special', 'blessed' and a 'blessing on the family'. For other cultures people with disabilities may be seen as a mark of shame and something to be hidden away as this may be interpreted as punishment for misdemeanours in previous lives. It is always best to take the lead from the individual and the family and, if possible, listen to what they have to say first. They may not be correct or always right but it will help the nurse to understand and work with the individual and their family in a more appropriate way.

When considering verbal skills, the actual words used must be considered. Nurses need to choose their words carefully so that they match the patient's ability to understand them. This is particularly important when giving information to patients. It is very easy to slip into jargon, especially when explaining a complex situation which may only be partially understood by the general population. The possibility for misunderstanding is increased when either party does not have English as a first language, and is even more likely when neither speak English fluently. Even when English is spoken fluently, accents, dialects, euphemisms, colloquialisms, abbreviations and acronyms (see Chapter 3) can obscure understanding to the point where the patient may be disappointed, alienated or, worse still, their healthcare may be compromised.

Physical disability

Many people in society live with a physical disability. People who have limbs missing – paraplegics, hemiplegics and quadriplegics – have individual needs and may experience difficulties or barriers when communicating their health needs and feelings. They may not be able to use the same non-verbal expressions as able-bodied people and nurses need to be aware of these difficulties. There may also be logistical issues – for example, a high counter that restricts the ease with which a person using a wheelchair or someone of short stature can talk to a receptionist.

Activity
- Try sitting in a wheelchair for an hour in the corner of a hospital waiting room. Write a reflection on how this experience made you feel. Note how many people spoke to you, looked at you or avoided you.
- Before you started nursing, how did you regard people in a wheelchair?

Vignette   Recognizing pain – physically and psychologically
Fred is 83 and has been receiving palliative treatment for eight years for prostate cancer. He lives with his 85-year-old wife Edna who has chronic obstructive airways disease and mid-stage Alzheimer's. Fred still drives an automatic car and has an electric scooter for getting around his garden. In the house he uses a frame and sometimes a wheelchair. Fred can usually manage about 10–20 steps unaided but must then rest. Both he and Edna are hard of hearing. Fred still tries to do as much as he can in his garden despite his difficulties. While standing on the back of a pick-up truck to cut the hedge he slips and falls to the ground. A neighbour hears Fred calling for help and on finding him calls for an ambulance. On arrival at A&E Fred is in a lot of pain, cannot hear what anyone is saying to him and is very worried about what has happened to Edna. He is shouting and calling out. Following X-rays, he is told he has broken nothing but is taken to

the ward because he is in so much pain. His clothes are a bit smelly and torn and he has not had a shave.

The nurses tell him off for disturbing the other patients and give him paracetamol. Later that night Fred's pain is so bad he insists on a doctor being called, who examines Fred and diagnoses three broken ribs. A morphine drip is started but Fred is still calling out in pain many hours afterwards. The nurses laugh at Fred and tell him he sounds like a woman giving birth and to stop making such a fuss. In the morning, Fred's daughter arrives to find Fred crying, which she has never seen before. The nurses are called and it is discovered Fred's drip has come undone in the bed, which is very wet, leaving Fred distressed and still in considerable pain.

Activity

- Reflect on the above situation and write down what you would have done differently.
- Before you read the next section, write down how you think Fred might be feeling.

Patient perspective

'I was in so much pain, nobody would listen – I just wanted to die but I was so worried about Edna. I could not understand that doctor or what he was saying – I tried to tell him it was my back that I fell on and hurt but he just kept fiddling with my front. When I got to the ward the nurses were very rough with me and kept laughing – how could they be so cruel to keep laughing at my pain? I thought I would die, then another doctor came and he was kind and said I had broken ribs and told the nurse to give me a drip or something. They said I was making more noise than women giving birth – I felt ashamed. If I ever get out of here I will never come back again – only if I am dead first. I spoke to Edna on the phone just now and she is mad at me for leaving her alone – she thinks I have gone to football and not come home.'

Activity

- How do you think Fred was treated? Was he treated with dignity, respect and compassion? How could his care have been bettered?
- What communication skills could/should have been used?
- What should happen now? Try drawing up a person-centred plan.
- Is compassion something we all have, or do we have to learn it? Do you think Fred was exposed to 'barriers to doing' or 'barriers to being' or both?

In Fred's case above, you may have considered issues such as the apparent pre-conceptions made about Fred and the dismal communication skills demonstrated by some of the staff 'caring' for him, regarding both his level of pain and his level of anxiety. Furthermore you may have noted the lack of dignity, respect and compassion afforded to Fred, while completely disempowered in the hospital environment.

The above scenario can also be used to consider communication issues in older people as well as those with limited mobility.

Older people

Older people often find it difficult to reveal personal information to others, particularly to a much younger person, even if it is a nurse. It is important for the nurse to pay special attention to communicating their respect for the patient – for example, by asking how they would like to be addressed, rather than assuming that first names are acceptable. Nurses need to ensure that any help given is really needed and wanted. Pressure of work often means that time is short, however, building a rapport with an older patient requires time and an air of being unhurried, while at the same time being efficient. It is useful to remember that dentures and hearing aids may be regarded as embarrassing signs of ageing by some older people.

Standards of care for older people have been at the centre of recent debates concerning dignity and compassion in nursing and the NMC has launched its new guidance (NMC 2009). The guidance sets out what older people expect when receiving care and provides a framework for nurses to challenge poor standards of care.

Activity
- Download a copy of the NMC (2009) document, *Care and Respect Every Time* from the NMC website.
- Review the content and think about how you can apply these principles in your everyday practice.

This would be a useful activity to discuss with your peers, and you may wish to record your discussions to add to your portfolio.

Reflection point
Think about an older person you have encountered as a patient.

- Were you anticipating any difficulties as you approached them?
- What difficulties did you actually experience?
- What strategies did you employ?
- Think about your personal preconceptions when working with different groups of people such as older people, people with a learning disability, those with mental health issues and those with sensory deprivation.

You may have found yourself surprised as to how fit and active some older people are. This reminds us that every person needs to be treated with dignity and respect and according to their needs and not their chronological age, disability or diagnosis.

Sensory deprivation

There are approximately 24,000 deaf-blind people in Britain (Butler 2004) but this does not include many elderly people who do not bother to register, as they accept this as a consequence of growing old. Stigma is often associated with sensory impairment and people complain they are often spoken to as if they are children, dim-witted and can do nothing for themselves.

Activity
- Tie a blindfold around your head and sit quietly for five minutes – try to time this without looking at a watch and see how long you actually think five minutes is with no eyesight.
- Now cover your ears with mufflers and do the same exercise.
- Now get a colleague to try to give you a drink with the blindfold and ear mufflers on without saying anything.
- Think about how this made you feel, what your emotions were.
- How could you help someone feel safe and empowered in this situation?

Vision loss

Sight problems affect people across the age spectrum, from all walks of society and cultures. People with vision loss, either complete or partial, will learn different ways to undertake activities of living, and their communication needs should be considered as part of this. When communicating with a blind person, it is important to relax and not feel you have to behave differently. If possible you should avoid trying to talk in a noisy environment as it may cause distraction and be difficult for the person to hear what is being said. You should speak normally and continue to use normal gestures and words. Body language can affect the tone of your voice and this will convey meaning in the conversation. A blind person may not always realize when a conversation is being directed to them, so it is important to use their name when talking within a group, and to introduce other people present. When you have finished speaking, do not leave without telling the person you are going (Vision Australia 2007).

Hearing loss

Royal National Institute for Deaf People (RNID) provides a number of resources and information for the deaf and hard of hearing. Hearing may also be impaired by tinnitus. Loss of hearing is not an 'obvious' disability, in that another person may not immediately realize that the person they are talking to may be experiencing hearing loss, as there may not be anything to see. Healthcare workers need to be mindful of the Disability Discrimination Act (1995) which requires equality of access to all areas of life for those with any type of disability. It requires that reasonable adjustments are made to enable people with disabilities to access a service and can apply to the way a service is offered (DirectGov 2009).

Reflection point
Think about your last placement.

- How were the needs of people who are deaf or hard of hearing accommodated?
- What facilities or tools can you use to communicate with people who have a hearing impairment?

RNID makes a number of recommendations to support healthcare workers in communicating effectively with people with hearing loss:

- asking patients for their preferred method of communication and ensuring this is recorded;
- ensuring there is sufficient time in the appointment;
- use of a display board to call patients into their appointments/make announcements;
- providing support, such as a sign language interpreter;
- providing equipment such as an induction loop;
- ensuring staff are aware of and can use 'text relay', which facilitates communication between text phones and telephones;
- always facing the patient;
- ensuring that at least one staff member has received basic deaf awareness training – preferably more than one.

It is important to remember that many people with varying degrees of hearing loss rely on lip-reading and/or facial expressions to fully understand what is being said. Further guidance from RNID (2009) suggests the following useful advice.

- Even if someone is wearing a hearing aid it doesn't mean they can hear you. Ask if they need to lip-read.
- If you are using communication support always remember to talk directly to the person you are communicating with, not the interpreter.
- Make sure you have face-to-face or eye-to-eye contact with the person you are talking to.
- Make sure you have the listener's attention before you start speaking.
- Speak clearly but not too slowly, and do not exaggerate your lip movements.
- Use natural facial expressions and gestures.
- If you are talking to a deaf person and a hearing person, do not just focus on the hearing person.

- Do not shout. It is uncomfortable for a hearing-aid user and looks aggressive.
- If someone does not understand what you have said, do not keep repeating it. Try saying it in a different way instead.
- Find a suitable place to talk, with good lighting and away from noise and distractions.
- Check that the person you are talking to can follow you. Be patient and take time to communicate properly.
- Use plain language and do not waffle. Avoid jargon and unfamiliar abbreviations.
- If there is no response, try a light touch on the arm and leave your hand there so the person can feel it.
- If the person does not want to communicate with you, they may pull away. Respect this and try again later.
- If you get no response, try taking the person's hand and drawing a capital letter of the alphabet (block writing) which is often used by deaf-blind people to spell out words.
- Remember to respect cultural differences and work with the whole family.

Dual sensory impairment

The prevalence of sensory disability increases with age, and sometimes both sight and hearing disabilities are present, resulting in a complex disability. There is a high rate of under-detection of sensory impairments, many of which can be treated. Sensory disabilities are often associated with challenging behaviour, often because people are unable to explain their needs. Remember that communication is more than just speech. There are many other ways to communicate, and listening and observing are critical. The barriers to good communication are often to do with the person on the receiving end of the communication rather than the originator of the communication. People on the receiving end need to be *alert, aware, attentive*, with the right *attitude* and the ability to respond *appropriately*.

Sensory problems can be congenital and may also progress or be acquired later in life. Services must be flexible and understanding enough to work with people who have disabilities and special approaches may be required for people who do not cooperate with the usual methods of assessment. Many people with sensory disabilities have other disabilities and complex needs. People with learning and sensory disabilities may need access to systematic teaching approaches which have been shown to develop the abilities of even the most severely disabled individuals. Such programmes not only improve the quality of life through personal development but may also have positive effects in reducing distress, as shown in reduction of challenging behaviours such as self-injury (DH 1998). Common-sense tips on approaching someone with dual sensory loss based on those recommended by Butler (2004) are:

- gently approach the person from the front or side so that if they have vision they can see you;
- try using clear speech first, speaking closely to the person, but do not shout in their face.

Vignette   'Can't you understand what I'm saying?'

Mr Josef Jankowski, aged 80, lived alone independently, despite the loss of his sight at age 60 following treatment for cancer. As he got older, his hearing also deteriorated. English is not Mr Jankowski's first language, although he has lived in England for over 50 years. Deterioration in his health led him to be admitted onto a medical ward, and he was feeling rather disorientated and cross at being away from his own home. Mr Jankowski's son, Paul, advised the nursing staff regarding his father's sensory deficits and language barriers and explained that his father liked to be called Joe. He advised them to speak clearly into Joe's better ear, so that he would have the best opportunity to understand. During visiting time the next day, Paul observed a nurse shouting directly into his father's face and calling him 'Josef' in an attempt to communicate.

Activity

- Put yourself in Paul's shoes – how would you feel observing this?
- What strategies could be used to communicate with Joe more effectively?
- What could the staff do to ensure everyone understood the best way to approach and speak to Joe?

Patient perspective

Here is Mr Jankowski's view of the situation:

'I don't know quite where I am here . . . I don't know the way to the toilet and there are so many noises I can't make out what's going on. I want to go home.'

His son took this view:

'I explained to the nurses that my dad can't see and that his hearing is not that great – I know it's not always easy for him to understand what has been said first time and I'd told the staff that when he was admitted. I found it distressing to see how he had been approached.'

You may have considered issues such as the confusion that the unfamiliar environment might have created for Mr Jankowski, the background noise, lack of visual cues when being approached by staff and communication issues within the nursing team. Evidently the information about talking into Joe's better ear, and how he liked to be addressed, had not been shared effectively.

Environmental influences

Environmental influences can be considered in terms of developmental impact and also in terms of behaviour. Exposure to sudden changes in environment can cause significant stress for anyone, and especially for someone with communication difficulties, as with Mr Jankowski in the previous vignette. Change brings with it the fear of the unknown for many people, but for people who cannot understand what is happening to them, this can be terrifying, especially if they are experiencing pain. Consider the following vignette which concerns the needs of Bob, a man with sensory and physical impairment admitted to hospital for investigations.

Vignette   Bob's life

Bob is 58 years old, he is totally blind, does not use verbal communication but can make sounds. He spends most of his day in a wheelchair. Recently he has had bouts of unexplained vomiting, usually after eating food. He is admitted to the medical ward for close observation and further investigations. A nurse notices that Bob is parked up in a corner with his hands over his face and assumes he is being ignored and excluded, so the nurse decides to move Bob forward to the other side of the bed nearer to other people. The nurse does this without saying anything to Bob first. Bob begins to rock and make screeching sounds. The nurse tries to comfort Bob by putting her arms around him, which makes Bob even more agitated. Another nurse arrives on the scene and says, 'Don't worry abut him, he's blind and he's probably like that all the time.' Meanwhile Bob throws himself out of the wheelchair and onto the floor, and curls up, sobbing.

Activity

- How should blind people be approached?
- What are the possible alternative reasons for Bob's behaviour?

On observation it may seem that Bob is being ignored and excluded but attempts to bring him into the centre of the room to socialize result in extreme agitation. Often where people with disabilities are unable to express their needs due to compromised communication skills, they will use means that health professionals regard as 'challenging behaviour'.

In this case, an initial reaction and assessment by the nurse might have assumed that this is how blind people behave because it is a feature of their condition and goes with their disability. However, a full assessment of the behaviour given in the example above reveals that Bob previously shared his life on a ward with 40 other men over a 35-year period and was frequently subjected to abuse which included slapping, pulling off clothes, scratching and biting. Bob was terrified he was going to be attacked again and was trying to make himself invisible to protect himself from harm. Once he was put back in the corner he quickly calmed down.

Environmental factors can be the key, and include things like room size (too large and too many people in it, or too small and enclosed with no personal boundaries and space of one's own). Consider how you interact with a patient in a bay with the curtains drawn. While there is a semblance of 'physical privacy', all conversations can easily be overheard. Other factors include noise, smells, temperatures, furnishings, lighting and design suitable for people with physical and/or sensory disabilities.

<hr>

Reflection point
- Think about situations where you have reacted before finding out all the facts.
- Think about situations where you have experienced being at the mercy of someone else's misinformation or limited knowledge. How did this make you feel?
- Why do you think so many able-bodied people think people in wheelchairs cannot speak or do anything for themselves?

<hr>

It is important to remember to treat all people as individuals first, making the effort to find out as much as possible about them before considering healthcare delivery unless it is an emergency. Asking others (especially those who know the patient best) for help is not negotiable. Patient care will be compromised if nurses rely solely on their own observations and expectations, especially when dealing with patients who have communication difficulties. Nurses need to have a knowledge and understanding of the way in which external influences and past life events will have shaped the individual's response to their current situation.

Conclusion

The art of effective communication with all members of society is an essential nursing skill. Key issues concerning some of the most vulnerable members of society have been considered here and it is important that nurses recognize the impact that disability may have on effective communication.

- Barriers to communicating and consulting with patients can occur at the most unexpected times and from the most unexpected people.
- Nurses can do much to negate and change the attitudes of others, but they must sometimes change their own attitudes first.
- By developing knowledge, self-awareness and insight, nurses can avoid prejudgement of their patients.
- Nurses must consider the impact of disability in the widest sense on their daily practice and strive for improvements in how they approach patient care.

References

Brooke, J. (1999) Derided we fall, *Nursing Times*, 95(4): 28.
Butler, S.J. (2004) *Hearing and Sight Loss – A Handbook for Professional Carers*. London: Age Concern.

Cooper, S.A. (1997) High prevalence of dementia among people with learning disabilities not attributable to Down's syndrome, *Psychological Medicine*, 27(3): 609–16.

DH (Department of Health) (1998) *Signposts for Success*. London: The Stationery Office.

DirectGov (2009) *Disabled People*, www.direct.gov.uk/en/DisabledPeople/HealthAndSupport/YourRightsInHealth/DG_4001074 (accessed 5 September 2009).

Dore (2010) Dyslexia fact sheet, www.dore.co.uk.

DRC (Disability Rights Commission) (2006) *Equal Treatment: Closing the Gap. A Formal Investigation into Physical Health Inequalities Experienced by People with Learning Disabilities/Mental Health Problems*, http://83.137.212.42/sitearchive/DRC/library/publications.html. Unavailable.

Mencap (2007) *Death by Indifference: Following up the 'Treat Me Right' Report*, www.cpaa.org.uk/node/320.org.uk (accessed 25 March 2010).

NMC (Nursing and Midwifery Council) (2008) *The Code: Standards of Conduct, Performance and Ethics for Nurses and Midwives*, www.nmc-uk.org.uk (accessed 11 March 2010).

NMC (Nursing and Midwifery Council) (2009) *Care and Respect Every Time: New Guidance for the Care of Older People*, www.nmc-uk.org/aArticle.aspx?ArticleID=3607 (accessed 18 March 2010).

Prothero, S., Ashby, S. and Taylor, S. (2009) *Primary Care*, in A. Glasper, G. McEwen and J. Richardson (eds) *Foundation Studies for Caring*. Basingstoke: Palgrave.

RNID (Royal National Institute for Deaf People) (2009) Communication tips for hearing people, www.rnid.org.uk/information_resources/communicating_better/tips_for_hearing_people/ (accessed 28 August 2009).

Thomas, C. (1999) *Female Forms: Experiencing and Understanding Disability*. Buckingham: Open University Press.

Vision Australia (2007) *Communicating Effectively with People Who are Blind or Vision Impaired*, www.visionaustralia.org.au/info.aspx?page=822 (accessed 28 August 2009).

7 Communicating in challenging situations

Mary Northrop

The daily practice of healthcare can present us with any number of challenging situations, and there are a range of communication tools which can be used to cope with these. Precipitating factors are considered here, and strategies offered to help prevent or minimize their occurrence. Theoretical perspectives include assertiveness skills, transactional analysis, behavioural approaches and ego defence mechanisms. Scenarios from both the practice and academic settings illustrate the use of problem-solving options. The approaches used are applicable to a wide range of situations in the daily practice of healthcare and other areas. Underpinning all of the scenarios is the importance of maintaining the dignity of all involved and ensuring respect for each other (see Chapter 3).

Learning outcomes

By the end of this chapter you should be able to:
1 Describe the factors that lead to challenging situations.
2 Understand how our own communication skills may diffuse or escalate situations.
3 Describe different techniques for communicating effectively in challenging situations.

Introduction

In both our professional and personal lives, challenging situations may occur that test an individual's effectiveness when communicating. These situations are influenced by personalities, values and beliefs, life experience and the context of events.

Every communication situation entered into depends on a number of factors as to whether that situation is perceived to be, or becomes, challenging. Previous chapters have addressed the issues of principles of communication and barriers. One person's perception of the same event may be different from another's. They may consider the interaction was positive while the other person may consider they have been bullied or their opinions not listened to.

Reflection point

Think about a situation where you felt you have not had your opinion listened to or have felt bullied – for example, making a complaint to a large organization via a call centre. Or imagine you are a waiter in a restaurant and a customer clicks his fingers to attract your attention.

- How did it make you feel?
- How can both parties resolve the resulting mixed messages in future encounters?

Attribution theory

Factors influencing individuals' perceptions of an encounter include attribution theory (developed by Weiner 1980, cited by Gross 2001). Problem interactions are explained through attributing the behaviour of others to internal causes, such as the individual's character or personality, or to external factors, including the situation they find themselves in or other distractions.

Along with attributes there are certain expectations we have of individuals, which are linked to social settings and roles. Goffman (1959) explored the concept of 'dramaturgy': people as social actors, who perform roles in relation to those they are interacting with. Within this theory, there are expectations of interactions in certain settings. For example, when visiting the GP there is a pattern of communication which resembles the script of a play. The GP will ask certain questions, probably perform an examination and prescribe a course of treatment. The patient will respond by giving details of their complaint. Neither the GP or the patient would expect to have a conversation about a film they had both seen.

The preferred option is always to prevent a challenging situation arising. In healthcare work, there are a whole range of situations where clients and their families may feel powerless and reliant on the healthcare professional to see them through a crisis. This will partly be due to the health problem they are experiencing but also because they are unfamiliar with the processes and procedures. By recognizing this, healthcare workers can give clients appropriate information throughout their care, listening to their concerns and dealing with these effectively and in a timely matter.

Reflection point

Think about a situation where you or one of your relatives or friends needed to access healthcare. This may have been via an outpatient clinic, A&E or other setting.

- How did the person and their accompanying relatives feel?
- How did the staff working in the healthcare environment act to ensure that effective communication occurred?

> - If anything was lacking or there were factors that may have led to confusion, anxiety or confrontation, how could the staff have improved the patient's and their family's experience?

Patient perspective

'I received a phone call saying I needed to go to the hospital as my husband had fallen off a ladder. On arrival, I was shown to the waiting room but no one seemed to know what was happening. They promised to find out and come and talk to me but after waiting an hour I had to ask again. All the staff avoided eye contact and I was left wondering what was going on, which at best was very irritating and at worst very worrying. When a staff nurse finally came to talk to me, she explained they were waiting for the orthopaedic surgeon. If I had been told this I would have been less worried.'

Another patient had a different type of experience:

'I had to attend my doctors' surgery as I had had a blood test and the results were higher than they should be. The doctor was new to the surgery and we had not met before. She came out to the reception area to take me to the consultation room, introduced herself and throughout the consultation asked my opinion and listened to what I had to say. She also took her time and I went away with my questions answered. This was much better than when I saw one of the other partners who rang through to reception and you had to find your own way to the consultation room. He also kept looking at the computer screen rather than me and did not ask my opinion.'

Your own reflections may have considered the level of anxiety regarding the reason for accessing healthcare. As in the two examples above, factors such as waiting times and the information made available by staff will have contributed to the experience, along with the initial communication with staff and how you were greeted. Other factors would include the knowledge and prior experience of the individuals as well as their ability to cope with and understand the situation. Consider the following team perspective from Michael, a healthcare assistant, concerning a child admitted for surgery.

Team perspective

'The porter arrived on the ward to transport Rosie to theatre and introduced himself to her and mum. The nurse in charge checked Rosie out by asking mum all the important questions on the pre-op check list in the notes while I tried to get Rosie on the bed ready to go. When I asked her to get on the bed she refused and started crying and looked frightened. I tried to calm Rosie down by asking in a calm manner what was wrong and gave her time to answer me. She said that she did not want to be put to sleep because this is what happened to her dog Ben when he was put to sleep two weeks prior to this event.'

Reflection and critical incident analyses

Past experiences can also act as effective learning tools, through the use of reflection or critical incident analysis. In order to increase understanding of one's
own skills and areas needing development, the use of reflection on a situation
can be beneficial. There are a wide range of models of reflection which enable the
practitioner to learn from a situation in relation to what worked well and what
could have been done differently (Gibbs 1988; Johns and Graham 1996; Driscoll
2007).

Critical incident analysis is often used after a specific event in order to look at
what was effective and what could have been done differently. For example, if a
patient has a cardiac arrest, those involved can review the event, drawing on their
perception of what happened and the written notes of the sequence of events.
Positive aspects can be incorporated into future practice and lessons learned from
what was not effective.

In examining a challenging situation the analysis can incorporate the 'ABC' approach:

- *Antecedents* – what led up to the situation?
- *Behaviour* – what those involved did.
- *Consequences* – the consequences of the behaviour.

The following scenario explores this in more depth.

Vignette   Managing aggressive behaviour
George is a patient on the ward. He is aged 73 and has a diagnosis of dementia.
He is confused and keeps trying to leave the ward to get home for his tea.
Derek, a student nurse, has been allocated to care for George. For the initial
part of Derek's shift he is able to distract George from leaving on a number of
occasions. However, this time, when he intercepts George as he is opening the
door of the ward, without thinking he tries to take George's hand off the door
handle saying, 'George, you can't leave the ward, you need to stay here.' George
responds by becoming angry and punches Derek.

Activity
- What do you think the antecedents to the event are for both George and
  Derek?
- Why do you think George reacted in the way he did?
- What could be done to prevent the situation from occurring again?

Using a critical incident analysis approach, the event can be examined and
lessons learned. Within the scenario the antecedents for George are linked to his

dementia. George is convinced that he needs to get home for his tea. He is not orientated to time, place or person and therefore does not understand why Derek is preventing him from leaving. To him, Derek is a stranger and Derek's touching of his hand and close body proximity invaded George's personal space and was probably interpreted as an attack. For Derek, the antecedents may be that he has managed George's behaviour for a number of hours successfully but has become tired or frustrated with stopping George from leaving and is therefore less patient with George on this occasion. The consequences of Derek's behaviour was his being punched by George and George feeling threatened and becoming more agitated.

By examining the preceding events the effective communication with George when he was successfully diverted can be incorporated into the future management. Bowie (1996), in his seminal work on aggression and violence in the workplace, suggests effective communication approaches when dealing with aggression and violence in the work setting in order to diffuse the situation. Some of these are also appropriate when dealing with a patient who is confused and therefore at risk of being aggressive. Paraverbal methods are particularly important: calm tone, appropriate eye contact and respect for personal space prevent the patient from feeling threatened. Other approaches, particularly for patients with confusion, are orientating the individual to time and place: explaining that they are in hospital and who you are may help them to recognize where they are. A further tool for confused patients is to distract them from their course of action, for example by asking them to talk about their home rather than concentrating on their wish to leave the ward or by involving them in an activity. The Alzheimer's Society (2008) recommends acting on the content of the patient's statement rather than the behaviour. They state, 'If the person says, "We must leave now – mother is waiting for me", you might reply, "Your mother used to wait for you, didn't she?"'

Reflection point

Think about your placements and a time where you have needed to communicate effectively with a person who is confused and disorientated.

- What strategies did you use?
- Were they effective?
- Is there anything you would do differently next time?

The lessons learned from what went wrong can be used to manage George's behaviour better in future and to address how staff are allocated to care for him. One solution is to ensure that there is a rotation of staff, to prevent one person having to deal with the situation for a long period of time.

For Derek, the analysis of the situation should enable him to reflect on what was effective about his communication and help him to learn to recognize when he needs to seek help. More importantly, this will identify how to support Derek following the incident. Derek's own view of the incident is given below.

Team perspective

'My initial reaction was of shock and then anger that a patient had punched me. This was rapidly followed by feelings of guilt when I realized that I had caused this reaction by how I had approached George. After discussing the incident with my mentor I was more aware of how the actions I took could be interpreted by George. The invasion of George's personal space, the removal of George's hand from the door knob and my tone of voice and content of speech, could be seen by him as an attack. On reflection, I also realized I had, until that point, been successful in caring for George and needed to consider what was effective but also develop further skills. My mentor suggested I listen to some stories of clients with dementia on the Patients' Voices website. I found the story *The Real Malcolm* (Patients' Voices 2010) to be informative and it reminded me of the individual beneath the illness.'

Empowerment

The vignette below also looks at ineffective communication with a patient, but examines different theoretical perspectives linked to power issues within the clinical setting and how these may lead to a challenging situation for a student nurse.

Vignette   Bath time

Aapti, a second-year student, has been allocated a group of clients to care for. The staff nurse has specifically asked that she ensures that Mrs Templeman, who is 80, has a bath. When she approaches Mrs Templeman and explains what she wishes to do, Mrs Templeman refuses and becomes very upset. She accuses Aapti of suggesting that she smells.

Reflection point

Put yourself into Mrs Templeman's shoes.

- How do you think this encounter has made her feel?
- How can Aapti approach such a situation differently next time to achieve a positive outcome for the patient?

Patient perspective

'That young nurse marched up to me and said "Come on, time for your bath!" She didn't ask whether I wanted one and she seemed to be suggesting that I smell. I had a bath yesterday and I didn't want another one today. I also don't like people bossing me about.'

There are a number of issues underlying this failure of communication. There are specific power issues in the scenario between Aapti and the qualified nurse, and Aapti and Mrs Templeman. Aapti has been asked to carry out the task by a qualified nurse and may be worried that she has been unable to do so. She may have been authoritarian with her communication and 'told' Mrs Templeman rather than ask her.

Using the theory of transactional analysis developed by Berne (1996), there are three ego states: the adult, the parent and the child. Aapti's approach may have led to a parent–child interaction rather than an adult–adult approach. This leads to a communication block as the interaction is not at the same level. The client may have underlying issues regarding her care to date and previous experience, which make her reluctant to have a bath, or she may have reacted to Aapti's parental approach by taking on the child role in the interaction.

Successful communication relies on both parties adopting an adult–adult style in the transaction. However, Aapti's approach could have been using the adult mode but Mrs Templeman's reaction could still be that of the child. The patient may feel disempowered by being in a hospital setting and may be coping by unconsciously projecting their own thoughts and attributing them to the healthcare worker.

Ego defence mechanisms

Sigmund Freud's seminal work, *The Ego and the Mechanisms of Defence* (1936), developed the concept of the id, ego and superego, theorizing that individuals use unconscious mechanisms in order to protect their ego. Wrycraft (2009: Ch. 13) presents a summary of the use of ego defence mechanisms. These mechanisms are employed unconsciously by individuals to protect themselves from anxiety and stress. They act as coping tools and protect the individual from feeling inadequate or worthless. They include:

- denial;
- displacement;
- projection;
- rationalization;
- repression;
- regression.

Reflection point

Situations such as the 'bath time' vignette above are not unusual. Think of a recent communication with a patient or a member of staff, where the interaction did not go as intended. Apply the concept of transactional analysis.

- Which ego states were present in the interaction?
- What underpinning factors could have influenced the interaction?
- What could be done differently to aid the creation of an adult–adult interaction?

Conflict resolution

The next vignette is more complex, in that a number of people are involved and, as with a real-life issue, part of diffusing the situation includes taking into consideration the perceptions of the event from the different participants. The vignette will be used to explore communication approaches that may be effective.

Vignette   'Where's my bag?'

Cynthia, a student nurse, is working in the ward office when she hears a patient, Talib, shouting at someone. When she investigates, one of the other patients, Lily, is accusing Talib of stealing her bag and is insisting on going through his locker to locate the bag and take it back. Talib insists that he has not done this and is becoming angry at both the invasion of his property and the accusation.

Activity

How might your perception of the event described in the vignette differ in the following contexts?

Type of ward

a)   A children's ward
b)   A mental health unit for the care of the elderly including clients with dementia
c)   An acute unit for mental health
d)   An emergency assessment unit
e)   A residential care unit for clients with learning disabilities

Participants involved

a)   Talib is aged 10 and known to play practical jokes on the other children
b)   Talib is aged 75 and has been admitted for assessment for depression; Lily is aged 78 and has Alzheimer's disease
c)   Talib is aged 28 and was admitted due to an alcohol and drug problem; Lily is a housewife aged 45 who has been admitted due to paranoia
d)   Lily is aged 73 and has been admitted in a confused state; Talib is 55 and has been admitted for investigation of chest pain
e)   Talib and Lily are both residents and were going out together; they have recently split up because Talib met someone else

There are a number of considerations regarding this latest vignette.

• Two clients are involved, both of whom will consider themselves to be the injured party. The context of the situation may influence how Cynthia reacts and may bring into play her own attitudes and, in some of the situations, prejudices.

- The nurse's role is to diffuse the situation and try to establish what is happening.
- As Cynthia is a student, her first action should be to get help from other staff members. The second action should be to separate the protagonists but to take into account the fact that both individuals need support.
- How the individuals are separated may depend on a range of factors. Who is the easiest person to remove from the area?
- Cynthia's own body language and tone of voice need to communicate a non-judgemental approach and calmness so that neither of the protagonists perceive her as taking sides.
- As Lily is invading Talib's space then it is preferable to move her from the vicinity if this is possible.
- Verbally explaining to Lily what is being done and why, and ensuring she understands that she is being listened to and her complaint is being taken seriously is essential regardless of the context or age.
- In Lily's case the use of touch may be applicable. Bowie (1996) suggests that the use of touch at the right time is calming and useful for clients who are frightened, but must be culturally appropriate.
- Talib also needs to be reassured that his viewpoint is as important and time should be provided to help him calm down. In the emergency assessment unit scenario this is a priority due to the possible underlying health problem.
- Recognizing that Talib is angry and acknowledging his anger can validate his response, which will allow him to begin to calm down (Faulkner 1998).
- Listening to Talib's viewpoint is important, as is informing him of any further actions that may be taken.

Working with colleagues

The preceding vignettes have focused on incidents involving patients or clients. This part of the chapter addresses situations that are more specific for student nurses both in practice and academic settings. The theories applied include assertiveness and conflict resolution, including negotiation.

The next vignette addresses a common occurrence in the classroom setting.

Vignette   'Quiet please!'
Georgina was attending a lecture at the university and was finding it difficult to hear the speaker due to two students behind her talking about what they were going to do that evening. What can she do about this? Consider the consequences of each action you suggest.

There are a number of factors to consider from Georgina's point of view.

- Is this the first occasion this has occurred with the same individuals?
- Does Georgina know the two students and feel confident to talk to them about the issue?

- Is she able to talk to them at this point?
- Would it be easier to move seats (if possible) and not confront them regarding their behaviour?
- Are other students disturbed by their talking and can they assist her?
- Should this be Georgina's responsibility or that of the lecturer?

Along with these questions, Georgina will also be drawing on her past experiences of similar situations and their outcomes. There is not necessarily a correct answer in this scenario and you may think of other alternatives. If Georgina moves seat, this is a short-term solution and may not address the problem. If she confronts the students about their talking the outcome may be positive in that they stop talking and apologize or they may resent this and continue. It will depend on how Georgina phrases and delivers her communication and how they interpret that communication. Kennedy (2008) outlines the importance of how we use tone of voice, language, body posture and other communication tools to communicate in an assertive manner and not a passive or aggressive way.

If Georgina asks the lecturer to deal with the situation, this is also not straightforward. The lecturer can act as a mediator and allow both parties to express their point of view, but this is not easy to do in the middle of a large lecture. Meeting afterwards is a possibility but this relies on Georgina gaining the cooperation of the other two students to stay behind. The lecturer may be able to monitor disruptions in future lectures and set ground rules to be followed. One of the overriding issues is that students are adults and need to take responsibility for their own behaviour.

Below is Georgina's account of how she actually dealt with the situation.

Team perspective

'I initially moved seats so I could hear the lecture as I did not want to miss anything or add to the talking by starting a conversation. As I knew the two students quite well I decided that I would talk to them afterwards even though I felt anxious about this. I spoke to them outside and explained that I had difficulty hearing because they were talking through the lecture. I explained that I needed to hear what was said as the subject was one I was struggling with and needed to understand for the assignment. They responded that they had not realized their talking was disturbing others and would try to talk more quietly next time. On reflection, by taking the approach that *I* had a problem meant I was not being assertive and I needed to point out that talking more quietly was still not appropriate.'

Negotiation and conflict resolution

The next vignette examines a group situation which is linked to conflict resolution and negotiation techniques.

Vignette   Group activity

Your current module requires a group presentation as part of the formal assessment. Your group of four meet and discuss how to divide the work between you and arrange to meet again the following week. At the set time, one of the group does not attend and has not contacted anyone to explain why. When they do make contact they state that they did not turn up because they felt the group was not listening to them and had given them the least interesting task to do.

Reflection point

Think about some of the times you have been asked to participate in group work.

- How do you feel about working in a group? Is this something you enjoy, or do you sometimes feel you are not listened to as part of a group?
- What strategies can you utilize to work effectively in a group?

Communication within a group relies on all members being able to say what they think in relation to a set task. One of the fundamental aspects of healthcare is the ability to work in teams to deliver care effectively. In this instance there is the underlying assessment which places greater stress on successful teamwork (see Chapter 5).

Within challenging situations we may need to bring in negotiation in order to achieve a satisfactory outcome for all involved (if possible). According to Spangle and Warren-Isenhart (2003: 21): 'Negotiation occurs when two or more people engage in problem-solving discussions designed to promote shared understandings, resolve differences, or engage in trade-offs that will be mutually beneficial'. In the above scenario, conflict resolution is required in order for all the students to be able to complete the assessment.

Linkemer (1999) describes some basic guidelines for conflict resolution, including the provision of a safe environment for all parties, that all sides of the issue will be heard and that common objectives exist to allow the conflict to be resolved. The last step is the provision of feedback following the meeting. She provides a 10-step format to achieve resolution. In the above vignette this would include the following:

- All of the members of the group *assume an open-minded approach*. If any of the group feel that there cannot be a resolution then the meeting may fail.
- The second stage is to *prepare for the discussion*. Each member needs to consider what they wish to say and how they can aid the meeting to be productive.
- The meeting is to resolve conflict and not to apportion blame. In this scenario, resolution to the conflict may need to be through a mediator, who may be another student who is respected by those involved. What needs to be avoided is a further rift if the individual feels the rest of the group is 'ganging up on

me' and that their viewpoint will not be heard. In this instance an independent mediator from outside the group, acceptable to all, would be preferable.

- The third stage is to *set the scene*, which includes both the setting in which the meeting will take place and setting out ground rules. Using Linkemer's guidelines the choice of venue needs to be neutral territory rather than at a student's house, and needs to ensure privacy for the discussion.
- The mediator will ensure that the room used is set up appropriately. For example, chairs in a circle allow for good eye contact and prevent students grouping together, creating a 'them and us' situation.
- The next two stages are *confirm your understanding of the issue* and *let the other person talk*. At the beginning of the meeting the mediator will remind everyone of the reasons for meeting and negotiate the setting of ground rules with the participants. This is essential to ensure constructive discussion and reduce the likelihood of drifting into verbal accusations.
- Each participant is then given an opportunity to express their views, with the mediator checking for understanding through the use of summarizing or para-phrasing. During this stage it is important that individuals are given equal time and consideration. The role of the mediator is to ensure this happens but also that what is said is constructive and does not drift into accusations or character assassinations.
- The next stages are *identify areas of agreement, state your position* and *talk through areas of contention*. Once all the viewpoints are heard, a summary of the issues is given and then the students will be asked to consider what issues they agree on, their own position and what they may be willing to change and what they are not.
- By identifying areas of contention negotiation may be possible through present-ing alternative solutions. This may involve compromise on both sides.
- The student who feels they have the least interesting task may reconsider if they understand the relevance and importance of their role. The rest of the group may accept that viewpoint and look at how the work can be redistributed to ensure all have a task that interests them.
- The last two stages are *if possible resolve the issue* and *follow through*. The decisions made can then be documented and agreed to by all present.

The other result of the meeting may be failure to resolve the conflict within the group and this should be considered as a potential outcome. However, the experi-ence of the process of conflict resolution and negotiation can be a valuable learning opportunity. An alternative resolution may be for the student who is dissatisfied to join another group.

Preventing a situation arising in the first place

When working in groups, particularly where assessments are linked to the output, a useful approach is to determine who will act as the chair and scribe. By setting up some of the principles of conflict resolution to prevent conflict this will aid in en-suring that all participants feel they are equally involved. Giving individuals equal time, the establishment of objectives and how consensus will be agreed may prevent later disagreements. The taking of minutes and summarizing decisions made at the end of the meeting allows individuals to agree or clarify any misunderstandings. Often, after decisions are made in a meeting, individuals may reflect back and wish to modify the agreed outcomes. By setting up communication between the group members, either online or face to face, any further issues can be discussed. The typing up of minutes and sending them to members of the group can also be a useful aide-memoire to what was agreed.

Assertiveness skills

The next vignette introduces the concept of assertiveness when communicating with others. Back and Back (1999: 1) describe what is meant by assertive behaviour. They define assertion as: 'Standing up for your own rights in such a way that you do not violate another person's rights. Expressing your needs, wants, opinions, feelings and beliefs in direct, honest and appropriate ways'.

They also describe two other types of behaviour: firstly, *non-assertion*, which is seen as 'Failing to stand up for your rights or doing so in such a way that others can easily disregard them. Expressing your needs, wants, opinions, feelings and beliefs in apologetic, diffident or self-effacing ways. Failing to express honestly your needs, wants, opinions, feelings and beliefs' (p. 2). Secondly, they describe *aggression*, which includes: 'Standing up for your own rights, but doing so in such a way that you violate the rights of other people. Ignoring or dismissing the needs, wants and opinions, feelings or beliefs of others. Expressing your own needs, wants and opinions (which may be honest or dishonest) in inappropriate ways' (p. 3).

When communicating using assertive techniques, the outcome is not the main issue, rather it is how the communication was handled. The person using assertive communication gets satisfaction from how they communicated with the others involved, rather than 'winning'. By being assertive there is more chance of getting your own needs met and feeling more confident in future interactions. Using non-assertive behaviour can lead to a lessening of self-esteem and may use more nervous energy in trying not to upset others. In some instances individuals may feel that by using aggressive behaviour they achieve what they want. However Back and Back (1999) suggest there is a related loss of respect from others. Cox (2007) provides guidelines on how to communicate assertively in situations involving the behaviour of colleagues. She suggests using the 'DESC' approach:

- *describe* the behaviour;
- *explain* the impact of the behaviour;
- *state* the desired outcome;
- *consider* the consequences of the behaviour if it does not change.

Cox also highlights that as individuals we shy away from situations because we do not wish to be confrontational. Following the model and rehearsing the conversation beforehand can aid the process.

Reflection point

How might the DESC model be employed by Georgina in the vignette on page 115?

Vignette   Learning contract

Michael is a student nurse who started the course six months ago. He has been on his current placement for a week and has been allocated Sally, the deputy ward manager, as his mentor. He is finding it difficult to meet with her to discuss his learning needs. He has arranged a time on two previous occasions which have been cancelled by Sally due to the ward being busy and her administrative role. He decides to try a third time and asks Ayira, a third-year student nurse, for advice. Ayira advises Michael to try again and be assertive to make sure his needs are addressed.

Activity

- How would you approach the above situation?
- How could Michael word his opening sentences to demonstrate an assertive approach?
- How would you apply the DESC approach?

In this instance Michael is doing his best to meet with his mentor in order to address his learning needs. He can understand why the mentor has been unable to meet with him but further delays will impact on his learning in the clinical setting. There are a couple of options available to him. His approach to the mentor needs to use assertiveness skills by stating his needs from his viewpoint but at the same time recognizing Sally's situation. Using these principles, Michael and Sally can address the situation together to find a solution. Both can express their own thoughts, feelings and concerns regarding the problem. By demonstrating understanding of each other's perspective they can move forward to find a solution. This may mean that both the mentor and student can arrange a time which is not likely to be cancelled, even if this is outside work hours. Michael can be proactive in relation to his learning needs by preparing a draft learning contract based on the module learning outcomes and competencies, using the help of the third-year student and his personal tutor or one of the ward staff. This can be given to Sally prior to the appointment to have a starting point for negotiation.

A further option would be to discuss with Sally the possibility of having a co-mentor who does not have the dual role that Sally has and therefore may be able to give time to Michael when Sally is busy. This would enable Sally to continue in the role and ensure that her expertise and skills are available to and valued by Michael.

For all of these options it is the way Michael communicates with Sally and her response that will ensure that both parties feel happy with the outcome. Finally, if this does not work then Michael needs to utilize the support available to him from the university or within the NHS Trust to resolve the situation.

Mentor responsibilities

It can be argued that Sally needs to be addressing this situation rather than Michael. Under the NMC *Standards to Support Learning and Assessment in Practice* (2006), mentors are responsible for ensuring that students' learning is facilitated. The document states the responsibilities of mentors (p. 17) and these include:

* organizing and coordinating student learning activities in practice;
* supervising students in learning situations and providing them with constructive feedback on their achievements;
* setting and monitoring the achievement of realistic learning objectives.

Sally would be aware of this and is not deliberately cancelling the appointments. In order for her to carry out the role, she needs to examine the factors that are hindering her performance by using problem-solving techniques. This may involve delegating the role to another member of staff or delegating other work to enable her to continue to mentor Michael.

Conclusion

A number of theories and approaches have been considered in this chapter, which may be used across a range of challenging situations. Development of the skills for preventing or diffusing situations occurs over time and often through trial and error. All situations involve individuals with a range of personalities and bring with them their own experiences, and no two situations are ever the same. However, it is important to take note of the following points:

* When dealing with challenging situations the context and those involved need to be taken into account.
* Recognizing when difficult situations may occur and preventing them is preferable to having to deal with an event.
* When prevention is not possible, there are a range of skills and approaches the individual can develop to apply to the situation.
* Underpinning dealing with challenging situations is the practitioner's need to develop effective communication skills and to be able to adapt within situations.
* Practitioners' development of skills is aided by the use of reflection.

References

Alzheimer's Society (2008) *Communicating*, fact sheet 500, www.alzheimers.org.uk/factsheet/500?gclid=CP3unNOzvpsCFVUA4wodiEucDw (accessed 5 July 2009).

Back, K. and Back, K. (1999) *Assertiveness at Work: A Practical Guide to Handling Awkward Situations*, 3rd edn. London: McGraw-Hill.

Berne, E. (1996) *Games People Play: The Basic Handbook of Transactional Analysis*. New York: Random House.

Bowie, V. (1996) *Coping With Violence: A Guide for the Human Services*. London: Whiting & Birch.

Cox, S. (2007) Good communication: finding the middle ground, *Nursing Times*, 37(1): 57.

Driscoll, J. (ed.) (2007) *Practising Clinical Supervision: A Reflective Approach for Healthcare Professionals*, 2nd edn. Edinburgh: Bailliere Tindall, Elsevier.

Faulkner, A. (1998) *Effective Interaction with Patients*, 2nd edn. New York: Churchill Livingstone.

Freud, S. (1936) *The Ego and the Mechanisms of Defence*. London: Chatto & Windus.

Gibbs, G. (1988) *Learning by Doing: A Guide to Teaching and Learning Methods*. Oxford: Further Education Unit, Oxford Brookes University.

Goffman, E. (1959) *The Presentation of Self in Everyday Life*. New York: Doubleday.

Gross, R. (2001) *Psychology: The Science of Mind and Behaviour*, 4th edn. London: Hodder & Stoughton.

Johns, C. and Graham, J. (1996) Using a reflective model of nursing and guided reflection, *Nursing Standard*, 11(2): 34–8.

Kennedy, S. (2008) Cool, calm and collected, *Nursing Standard*, 28(37): 64.

Linkemer, B. (1999) *Working with Difficult People: The Essential Guide to Thinking and Working Smarter*. London: Marshall Publishing.

NMC (Nursing and Midwifery Council) (2006) *Standards to Support Learning and Assessment in Practice*, www.nmc-uk.org/aDisplayDocument.aspx?documentID=1914 (accessed 12 April 2009).

Patients' Voices (2010) *The Real Malcolm*, www.patientvoices.org.uk/naoeol.htm (accessed 1 January 2010).

Spangle, M. and Warren-Isenhart, M. (2003) *Negotiation: Communication for Diverse Settings*. Thousand Oaks, CA: Sage.

Wrycraft, N. (ed.) (2009) *An Introduction to Mental Health Nursing*. Maidenhead: Open University Press.

8 Communication in learning and teaching

Paula Sobiechowska

This chapter discusses how successful learning and teaching depends upon effective communication skills. The chapter makes clear the complexity of the environment in which communication in the learning process occurs and highlights some of the factors that help and hinder our capacity to learn. There is an emphasis on understanding ourselves as learners and how this influences the way we work with the opportunities available to us. In taking this stance, the chapter promotes a reflective approach to learning that depends on a willingness to critically engage with others through constructive and purposeful dialogue. A series of vignettes and reflection points are intended to illustrate the themes discussed.

Learning outcomes

By the end of this chapter you should be able to:
1 Recognize learning opportunities as they arise and develop a reflective approach to maximize the learning.
2 Develop a structure for all teaching situations, even those that are impromptu and informal.
3 Describe various strategies for teaching and learning.

Introduction

Successful learning and teaching relies on good and effective communication. The quality of the experience is dependent upon a number of factors ranging from the context to the personal attributes of those involved. Self-awareness is critical to effective learning, teaching and communication; it illuminates our potential for learning and communicating as well as the limitations we may want to overcome. Some learning opportunities are obvious; others less so, but perhaps more enlightening than we imagine.

Communication at the heart of learning and teaching

Effective communication is at the heart of the learning enterprise, as learning and teaching are essentially communicative acts (Knewstubb and Bond 2009: 181). In order to learn something I have to be open to receive some kind of information – listening to another person, reading a document or observing a person, people or a situation. In effect I am receiving a range of stimuli from the external world. However, I still have to make sense of this information to learn something from it and engage in another communicative process – thinking about what the information might mean, communicating with myself through the language of my thoughts. This thinking is usually a 'sense-making' or reflective activity, as I try to understand my new experience in relation to what I know already. I probably need to draw on some other resources, not just my own thoughts. This might require some more reading or talking to others. So, my sense-making reflections become another form of communication, a further exchange of materials between myself and the world. Eventually, I might want to tell someone else about what I heard, read or saw and what I think it means. To share my experience and my ideas I have to find an effective and engaging way of communicating with others, thus shifting my position a little, from being a learner to being a teacher as I explain and analyse a phenomenon with others.

When I share my considered ideas with others they usually respond, either questioning or affirming my views. Our interaction will depend on a number of sociocultural factors, which will be highlighted later in this chapter, but the important thing is that during this interaction we will be 'making meaning' together. We can come to a shared or, sometimes, divergent comprehension of the subject or experience we are discussing. When this process occurs, between lecturers and students, mentors and students, within student groups, we all become teachers and learners. In entering into this kind of communication we go beyond 'content' and 'facts' and actually begin to create knowledge, which is really quite exciting. In thinking about learning and teaching as communicative acts, the possibilities become more far-reaching than might be apparent in our scheduled lectures or mentor supervision sessions.

Thinking about the possibilities described above, we can see that we do not have to be on a university course to learn new things, or to be in a position to teach others. In practical terms we are all likely to find ourselves occupying the role of learner and/or teacher and these roles are fluid, sometimes changing several times within the course of an interaction. For example, as a patient I may teach you something about living with a chronic condition or a terminal illness. As we interact, you, as a nurse, may teach me about the importance of remaining mobile or taking my medication as prescribed. We will both be learning and teaching, and at the core of our enterprise we will be communicating by talking and listening to each other. For us to learn and teach it is critical that our communication with each other is empathic, clear, purposeful, respectful and empowering. If either party feels diminished in the exchange, we will have been unsuccessful, with the possibility of 'mis-learning' or no learning having occurred. Consider the nature of communication and its purposes from the perspective of this patient who has just arrived on a ward from A&E.

Patient perspective

'. . . this mask is making it hard to breathe even though it's meant to help. Here comes the nurse. She is asking so many questions about how I live at home,

> whether I can walk, if I'm on my own – for the discharge plan, she says. I've only just arrived. And I'm not worried about my smoking, right now I'm worried about my family.'

As in establishing effective relationships in nursing practice (e.g. see McCabe 2004), learning and teaching requires an authentic engagement between the learner and teacher. Authentic engagement means that all parties actively listen and attend to each other, express and acknowledge feelings and are mutually respectful of each other. McCroskey *et al.* (2002: 387) make similar observations about effective communications between teachers and learners in their focus on the importance of 'non-verbal immediacy' – for example, the promptness and degree of eye contact, guiding or containing touch and/or proximity between teacher and learner. The genesis of these ideas, a holistic approach to the communicative endeavour in education, was probably first proposed by Carl Rogers, who was concerned with notions of 'congruence (realness), acceptance and empathy' (Smith 2004) in the teacher–learner relationship.

Reflection point

Think about a situation where you were trying to learn a new skill or teach someone else. For example, removing sutures, undertaking a catheterization or assisting on a drugs round.

- What went well in the situation and why? For example, was it because the instructions were clear, or the teacher was patient with a calm but authoritative approach?
- What did not go so well in the situation and why? For example, did you become overanxious and maybe could not hear what the teacher was advising or asking?
- Given these initial reflections, how could you prepare yourself for learning or teaching new skills another time?

Learning and teaching is a transactional engagement that involves the exchange of information, ideas and experiences. If the *exchange* can be further developed into an *exploration* then learning and teaching can be a collective sense-making process. Ultimately this might enable us to improve or change something, either ourselves or an aspect of our world (Freire 1972; Mezirow 1991).

The learning environment

Figure 8.1 illustrates the complexity of the learning environment as experienced by both learners and teachers. The placement or workplace and the university are separated only by a dotted line as they are connected. All settings are located in

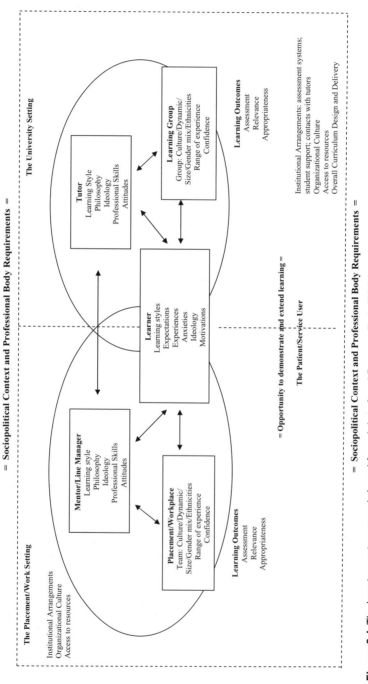

= Sociopolitical Context and Professional Body Requirements =

The University Setting

Tutor
Learning Style
Philosophy
Ideology
Professional Skills
Attitudes

Learning Group
Group: Culture/Dynamic/
Size/Gender mix/Ethnicities
Range of experience
Confidence

Learning Outcomes
Assessment
Relevance
Appropriateness

Institutional Arrangements: assessment systems;
student support; contacts with tutors
Organizational Culture
Access to resources
Overall Curriculum Design and Delivery

Learner
Learning styles
Expectations
Experiences
Anxieties
Ideology
Motivations

= Opportunity to demonstrate and extend learning =

The Patient/Service User

Mentor/Line Manager
Learning style
Philosophy
Ideology
Professional Skills
Attitudes

Placement/Workplace
Team: Culture/Dynamic/
Size/Gender mix/Ethnicities
Range of experience
Confidence

Learning Outcomes
Assessment
Relevance
Appropriateness

The Placement/Work Setting

Institutional Arrangements
Organizational Culture
Access to resources

= Sociopolitical Context and Professional Body Requirements =

Figure 8.1 The learning environment (adapted from Ashcroft and Foreman-Peck 1994)

the wider sociopolitical context that largely determines organizational policies and directives. In professional and vocational education everyone (students, mentors, consultants, managers and employers) is bound by the requirements and codes of practice of the professional bodies. Such policies, directives and codes of conduct connect the university with the world of practice but most importantly, for our purposes here, organizations and the university are connected through the learner and service user. This makes the learner the primary conduit for communication between the two systems and equally accountable to both organizations. The service user is central in the model as they provide the key site of the student's immediate learning and are also the focus of theoretical teaching delivered in the university. This centrality of the patient is made explicit in practice supervision and in the portfolio work and case studies that students are often required to produce for assessment.

Reflection point

To illustrate aspects of the relationship between the university and practice setting, think about a patient who has become a case study for you.

- How and why did you choose this individual? For example, because they were typical/atypical of a health condition, because discussions with your mentor/supervisor highlighted a particular aspect of the individual's situation?
- How well do the circumstances and experiences of the patient (e.g. diagnosis, care and treatment, outcomes) fit with the theoretical models discussed in the classroom or textbooks?
- Given these initial reflections, how might you incorporate your thinking about theory and practice in future assignment, presentation and portfolio tasks?

Figure 8.1 infers that the learner is subject to a variety of communications within both organizations, as indicated by the directional arrows, from tutors, mentors, managers and peers. If the learner does not pay sufficient attention to the various communications (e.g. policy and practice documents, academic texts, telephone calls, instructions, emails, lectures, group presentations) they could come unstuck. Also, if the communications to the learner are not clear the student could be disadvantaged. The diagram helps us appreciate the demands on the learner and the potential intensity of their experience. It highlights the need for learners and teachers to engage in a dialogue so that miscommunications and misunderstandings are minimized and shared meanings established. This may include mutual understanding of what is required, in terms of learning outcomes and standards to be achieved, documents to be completed, types of work to be undertaken and what to do if things start to 'go wrong'. These understandings and expectations are often managed through a learning contract, which might already be formatted by a learning programme. However, learners and teachers still need to bring their own 'stamp' to learning contracts to facilitate preferred learning styles, previous learning experiences and 'world views' or 'lifeworlds' (Barrington and Street 2008; Ekeburgh 2009).

Vignette   Negotiating a learning contract

Aashi is a second-year student nurse. The ward-based placements of the first year suited her as she was easily able to balance her family life and the course. She has now been placed in a community team and feels nervous. Aashi is aware that she will have to take more responsibility for her time management in the community, a setting that is more fluid than the familiar routine of the wards. Although she has transferable knowledge and skills, it has been recommended that she familiarizes herself with at least two other conditions that are managed in the community. There is documentation to be signed during the placement, but Aashi is not sure of her mentor's availability to supervise, monitor, assess and sign the paperwork. Tomorrow she meets her mentor to discuss the learning contract and placement experience.

Activity

- Consider the complexity of the learning environment and think about the roles and responsibilities of the learner and mentor in Aashi's situation.
- How can Aashi best prepare for the meeting with her mentor? What sort of role could she adopt in this meeting (e.g. should she be a more or less passive or active learner)?
- How could the mentor best prepare for the meeting? What would be a good approach to supporting her in the placement?
- What do you think might be the most important points to emphasize in the learning contract?

Once practice supervisors and students have established basic understandings, more complex, negotiated meaning-making can ensue and this is often concerned with the patient experience and local clinical practices. Learning regarding the service user and clinical environment is usually developed through discussions in both the university and practice settings. A student will discuss practice with clinical colleagues and also with university tutors and peers. In this discussion the learner has to manage the boundaries of confidentiality between the two spheres in which they are working and learning. The challenge lies in taking the experience from the practice environment into the learning environment, while maintaining the dignity, anonymity and confidentiality of service users and colleagues.

Vignette   Managing confidentiality

Geoffrey has just returned to university after a placement on a medical ward working with older people. To help him remember the practice issues, he kept a reflective diary and also took photos of ward situations and patients with his mobile phone. As well as bringing these to share with the tutor group he has included them in his e-portfolio as he thinks it lends authenticity to his work, an important aspect in portfolios. Geoffrey's peer group are very impressed with his materials and there is a lot of discussion, especially as a group member recognizes one of the patients from a previous placement. The conversation focuses on the details of this patient's situation. When the tutor arrives she stops the exercise and asks the group to stay behind over lunch.

Activity

- Thinking about the complexity of the learning environment and the relationships between all those involved, how do you understand what is happening in the last vignette?
- If you were the patient under discussion, or a relative, what might you think about this situation?
- How do the principles of the Nursing and Midwifery Council (NMC) *Code* (2008) help you to understand the issues raised in this scenario?
- As the tutor, how would you approach this situation with Geoffrey and the student group?

Understanding yourself as a learner

In both placement and university settings, learners and teachers have to establish relationships with each other. For the learner, this can be a particularly tricky negotiation, where the primary relationship is with powerful authority figures (the mentor or line manager and the tutor). This can feel intimidating, or might be viewed as a 'once in a lifetime' opportunity to work alongside an expert. As Fanthorne (2004: 53) notes, where confidence prevails students, as supernumeraries, are in a good position to 'approach those much higher up the company for advice or information'. Equally, relationships with peers operate on a continuum that encompasses the hugely enriching, through to the indifferent, and on rare occasions the damaging. In the context of professional learning it is always better to strive for positive and enhancing relationships with peers – these people are likely to be your colleagues, in one way or another, for the rest of your career. In reality professional worlds are often quite small.

All relationships are mediated through communication. The quality of communication between individuals and the types of relationships they have will be influenced by the personal histories and viewpoints of the various actors (Ekeburgh

2009; Knewstubb and Bond 2009). We bring a set of, sometimes hardly realized, expectations and assumptions into every encounter, which can be more or less helpful to the progress and outcome of relationships and the learning experience.

Vignette   Identifying and working with assumptions and expectations

Malik has joined the nursing programme expecting to learn a lot of factual information. The regular group work has come as something of a surprise – he hadn't expected to learn much from his 'peers'. He finds himself in a mainly female group. There is one other guy who he never sees outside of the group sessions. The 'girls' seem to have little in common with him and do not seem to concentrate on the group tasks. Every time they meet they have to share a reflective commentary on their practice experiences. Malik can describe what happens on the ward, but has difficulty offering a critical commentary as it would be disrespectful and disloyal to the staff in the placement. Consequently, Malik's contribution is brief and he mutters his way through his commentary. Thankfully, no one ever asks him any questions, they just get through the task as quickly as possible before talking about 'more interesting' things.

Activity

Think about the complexity of the learning environment and how relationships can be influenced by personal values and attitudes.

- How do you understand what is happening in this vignette?
- What could Malik do to improve the situation he finds himself in?
- What could an academic tutor or workplace/placement mentor do to help Malik learn in the group?

Malik's vignette highlights the importance of understanding yourself as a learner. As Cottrell (2005: 9) notes, it is important to be critically self-aware in terms of one's own personal and cultural 'baggage' in order to understand how we process information and experiences. As learners our experiences and expectations shape our engagement with others and therefore our learning. This becomes apparent when we reflect upon the following:

- the types of people with whom we feel most comfortable and to whom we can most easily talk;
- the types of information we can absorb;
- the ideas we can discuss openly and constructively.

For example, our community, cultural or ethnic experience and heritage may imbue us with strong beliefs about any number of matters – the role of women, the capacity of gender, the ethics or morality of abortion and care of the dying. Our experience and heritage may make it more or less challenging for us to explore honestly these topics with others. As Hanley (2009: 181) argues, whatever our world view, an openness to the exploration and examination of our professional experiences and academic and social discourses about the lives and rights of others is important for us to progress in our thinking and learning, and to enable us to be receptive to others. This critical engagement with ourselves does not necessarily mean we relinquish our beliefs or comprehension of the world, but that we develop a clearer, more informed understanding of those beliefs and comprehensions (Cottrell 2005: 9).

Vignette   Responding to professional and personal challenges

Alex, a third-year student, was coming to the end of his placement in the hospice, which he had found both challenging and uplifting. He was amazed at the resilience and bravery of the patients and their families, but was quite disturbed by the realities of the physical end of life, even with the administration of painkilling drugs. In the week before the placement ended a very unwell patient was admitted. The family were in agreement with the general treatment plan but were insistent on resuscitation in case of heart failure. They wanted everything to be done to save the life of the patient and would raise this point with all members of the team at every opportunity. Alex was involved in these conversations on a number of occasions and found them difficult as he thought the patient should be allowed to die peacefully. He said this to the family and a complaint was lodged. The complaint remains outstanding as Alex reaches the end of his course.

Activity

In the case of Alex, think about the complexity of the learning environment, and the range of values and attitudes that are brought into the setting by students, service users and practitioners.

- How do you understand what is happening in this vignette?
- How could Alex have managed the situation more effectively?
- What should have been happening in the placement setting to support Alex in his learning?

Alex has experienced something that challenges his firmly-held belief system. Long-established educational theorists, such as Freire (1972) and Mezirow (1991) argue that challenges to the self are central to authentic and transformative learning, that is, learning which makes a significant difference to our perspectives of the world and our relations and actions within it. Transformative learning is argued to occur when we are shaken out of our 'taken-for-granted' assumptions and practices, when we critically evaluate our new experience, derive new meanings from it and assimilate those meanings into new, refreshing perspectives. If we cannot openly explore what experiences might mean (from our own or others' perspectives), or what the limitations of a particular theoretical model might be (is it culturally or gender-biased, is it applicable only in particular circumstances, or is the evidence base small?) then it makes sense to ask, how are we learning? Notions of transformative learning are particularly important in professions such as nursing, which is located in a highly politicized and plural context. Every day, practitioners may find their understandings challenged by the introduction of a new policy or way of working, or by a patient who challenges or invokes stereotypes. Understanding and working with these challenges requires us to develop as reflective learners and practitioners. Beckett and Hager (2002: 139–46) raise a similar discussion in their theorizing of practice-based learning at work.

Reflection point
Think about your own assumptions and expectations.

- How do you respond when others express views or behave in ways that are different from what you expect? For example, do you dismiss or ignore them; become angry or defensive; or are you curious about how the other person sees things?
- How do you manage situations where your professional or personal perspectives are challenged? Again, do you dismiss or ignore the challenge or take time to think about and openly respond to any such challenge?
- Given these initial thoughts, how might you develop your capacity as a reflective learner and practitioner?

As well as identifying perceptual or attitudinal barriers to learning, it is helpful to be honest with others about more tangible obstacles to effective learning. Some are more apparent than others, such as hearing impairments, while others may only become evident over time. Dyslexia and dyspraxia, for example, may be identified quite late in a student's academic career. Such a diagnosis can be upsetting and put people 'off course'. However, the sooner a student and their teaching team know there is a need for different learning and teaching strategies the less problems arise for everyone (see Chapter 6).

Vignette   Managing your learning needs
Gillian was on the last module of her degree and assumed that the teaching team knew she had been diagnosed with dyslexia in the last semester. She was still trying to understand this diagnosis herself. It had come as a surprise – she just thought she did not understand much of the 'fancy talk' that went on in the university. Nonetheless, she was a bit anxious about getting into too much detail about what the diagnosis meant with anyone. As the tutors knew she thought they should come to her – she did not need to go around making a big deal

of it. Gillian managed to complete the final module but with a very low pass mark that left her feeling unhappy as she had worked hard. If what she had been drafting was not 'good enough', she wondered why the tutors had not talked it through with her more. She was left with a feeling of a lack of support from the tutor and teaching team, and she told them this in the evaluation at the end of the module. The module tutor was taken aback by her comments, because he had not known that Gillian was dyslexic.

Activity

Thinking about the complexity of the learning environment:

- How do you interpret what has happened in this scenario?
- What could Gillian have done to help herself as a learner?
- What could the academic team have done to help Gillian as a learner?

Reflection point

As a learner:

- Do you have any particular learning needs? For example, due to a condition such as dyslexia, or a hearing or visual impairment.
- Have you advised the teaching team (e.g. academic tutor, placement supervisor) about your learning needs? If not, why do you think that might be, and what would help you to tell them?
- What would be the most useful things for the teaching team to know about your needs?
- Can you propose an action plan that ensures you are enabled to meet your full potential?

Identifying learning opportunities

Edgecombe and Bowden (2009: 93) cite the work of Hart and Rotem to draw our attention to 'the difference between the clinical environment's complex social context and the more controlled classroom environment'. The curriculum design and skills of the facilitator can limit the role of the student to that of a passive recipient of knowledge from the expert teacher. Even in an enquiry-led approach, the academic model is often based on the incremental acquisition of knowledge, with the complexity of content and understanding building over time. Classroom learning opportunities are, superficially, obvious – lectures, group work exercises, tutorials – in which the release of information can be artificially controlled.

Conversely, the clinical environment confronts the learner with a range of social relations and a practice milieu out of which learning opportunities have to be sifted. Learning cannot be acquired in neat, pre-packaged units and emerge from the unpredictability of the day's work, irrespective of the student's level of study. Practice settings can be overwhelmingly busy and pressured, so that all the novice sees is a whirr of activity as colleagues move from one task to the next, without taking breath. At the other end of the spectrum a student might be left wondering what they should do, or even what it is they *are* doing, when each community visit only lasts ten minutes, and after the dressing has been changed there is only a bit of chat with the patient. However, it is useful to consider the same community experience from the perspective of this older person who is now confined to the sitting room of his home, as described in the next patient's perspective.

Patient perspective

'Well she doesn't stay for long, only seems like five minutes. Still, even though it's the pressure sores, and not very nice, the five minutes does make a difference. Sometimes I can be in a lot of pain, so it's reassuring when she comes. Can't talk about medical things to the carers or the meals-on-wheels man, can I? Not their business. Feel safer when she's been, she's made notes and reports back to the surgery, so I know I'll be all right.'

Although fluid and complex, the practice setting is not a 'free-for-all' learning experience. It is important for the mentor to exercise some control within the placement on behalf of the learner, identifying learning opportunities that enable students to demonstrate their competence in certain activities or practices. Equally, learning opportunities that can support students to meet more personalized goals (e.g. enhancing time management or organizational skills) should be negotiated. The balance between the requirements of the programme and the student's own learning needs is likely to be managed through a form of learning agreement (Barrington and Street 2008).

Generally, learning opportunities are likely to range from the formal through to the incidental. Unplanned, incidental experiences can be a source of rich learning when they are examined through a set of reflective questions (e.g. see Fish *et al.* 1991; Johns 1999; Beckett and Hager 2002).

Reflection point

Consider the learning opportunities below and decide how they might be located on a learning continuum of formal–informal–incidental. Make a note of your thoughts.

Learning opportunities

- Shadowing a drugs round
- Undertaking a patient observation

- Writing case notes
- Handover
- Accompanying a patient to theatre
- Working in the sluice room with a colleague
- Taking a personal history
- Joining a ward round
- Enabling a patient to maintain their dignity when using a commode on the ward
- Observing a consultant discuss a diagnosis with a patient
- Sitting with a bereaved family
- A supervision session

Any of the opportunities noted above could be understood as a formal experience. However, a number of them might arise, unplanned, during the course of a day's work. Payne and Scott (1982) devised a simple model for supervision in practice that can be adapted to frame our thinking about identifying and managing learning opportunities. Aspects of the model they describe are similar to the findings in more recent research into clinical supervision undertaken by Laitinen-Vaananen *et al.* (2007).

The formal/planned quadrant shown in Figure 8.2 represents the type of learning with which we are probably most familiar, where the learner and mentor agree a learning activity, such as accompanying a patient to the operating theatre. Ideally the learner and mentor will identify the student's pre-existing knowledge, perhaps documenting this in a reflective journal or mentor note. As a learning team they will identify what other knowledge the student requires before undertaking the task – this might involve further reading, talking to other patients or shadowing the

FORMAL

PLANNED	AD HOC
• Planned activities • Objectives agreed in advance • Agreed methods for reaching objectives • Direct supervision may occur in situ • Reflective supervision/debrief held after the activity/event	• Activity agreed and undertaken on the spot. • Direct supervision may occur in situ, or practices may be demonstrated/modelled • Reflective supervision/debrief held after the activity/event
• Routine activity: bathing; escort to the pharmacy; community visit; staff lunch • Conversational 'small-talk' • Professional conversation develops	• Activity arises out of the demands of the practice situation, or everyday routine • Discussion arises out of the situation as it unfolds; although direct supervision may not be evident modelling may be more apparent • Reflective supervision/debrief may or may not arise out of the activity/event

INFORMAL

Figure 8.2 A framework for clinical supervision (adapted from Payne and Scott 1982)

preoperative team in preparation. The mentor may directly supervise the student's practice by talking the student through the activity as it occurs. This type of learning opportunity might also be managed as an observation of the student's practice (with no guiding talk from the mentor, unless practice is unsafe). On completion the mentor and student will evaluate the success of the undertaking, with a view to identifying further practice development.

In all quadrants of the model the way the mentor works has the potential to demonstrate good practice for the learner. Such demonstration, or modelling, may be the most powerful mode of communication in the practice learning setting. It is likely to include the non-verbal presentation of the practitioner to a client – preferably calm, in positive control, attentive and concerned for the individual; hopefully, not too harassed, or in a hurry. Modelling will also encompass verbal communication – tone and pitch of voice, speed of speech and quality of content. The type of language used will demonstrate respect for the patient. These observations will inform the learner's view of professional practice and acceptable behaviour. Sometimes we are harassed or not performing as we should. Irrespective of whether practices within an event can be described as 'good', 'poor' or 'bad' it is valuable to re-examine the experience.

Reflection point

Think about a recent practice learning experience where you worked alongside a senior colleague.

- What sort of behaviours did your colleague demonstrate and from your observations what did you learn about effective communication? For example, to remain focused on the patient, to carefully repeat key information, to use touch to calm distress.
- Was there anything from this observation, or similar occasions, that seemed less than helpful in the interaction with the patient?
- Given these initial reflections, how might you continue to build your own communication skills through learning from your observations of others?

We tend to be less familiar with the informal/ad hoc learning opportunities that arise in practice. They can range from the dramatic, such as the sudden deterioration of a patient's health, to the seemingly mundane – for example, stopping to have a brief chat on the way to the linen cupboard. Some sort of debrief is likely to arise out of a patient's deterioration, possibly ongoing, as the team decide on interventions, or at a later stage when the team reflect back on what happened. It is important for learners to engage in these team debriefings, often located in this informal/ad hoc quadrant, as learning cannot be reliant on a mentor or one or two experts.

It is the 'small' unplanned encounters with patients and families that may go unnoticed and that are rarely the subject of our scrutiny. When service users choose to speak to us, and if we are receptive, then we can best meet their needs and learn something about how they cope with their circumstances. Listening to and understanding the patient and their family and carers is crucial. To heal, survive or die a good death individuals need their personhood to be respected and their psychological wellbeing to be upheld. If we overlook the communications of patients we potentially undermine the efficacy of all our clever scientific interventions. Consider, for example, the implications of the patient's experience in the next patient perspective.

Patient perspective
'. . . half-hourly observations, apparently, so they came and took my blood pressure, temperature and watched the machine every 20 minutes or so – sometimes more often if they were called away in the middle, or the machine started beeping. Never knew what that meant, but it was worrying. Never knew what any of it meant really, they didn't talk to me about how I was doing, just kept taking the measurements. Always felt I was taking up their time when I asked questions so in the end just decided to keep quiet, expect they'd have let me know if anything was seriously wrong . . .'

Developing reflective practice

In order to make sense of learning opportunities it is possible to use a format that, as already suggested:

• identifies what is already known and understood;
• explores the cognitive, affective, social and psychomotor aspects of practice for individuals (Beckett and Hager 2002: 30);
• identifies ways of 'filling the gaps' – for example, reading, observing others, talking to others with an enquiry-oriented purpose;
• identifies opportunities for developing practice – with or without supervision;
• evaluates the success of an intervention/interventions reflecting on what worked well or not, and why, through an ongoing reflective discussion.

Such an exploration also offers us the opportunity to look at the affective aspects of our learning. The feelings generated through learning experiences are worthy of our attention as we need to develop our capacity for emotional intelligence and emotional resilience. Emotional intelligence is central to working respectfully with the pains, sorrows, anxieties and hopes of the cared-for and of our colleagues. Equally, emotional resilience is necessary for us to manage for ourselves the feelings nursing practice and experience evokes.

The systematic approach being promoted here is informed by the ideas of experiential learning originally presented by David Kolb in 1984. The approach is also similar to the principles that inform action learning as described in the work of Reg Revans (WIAL 2009). The model is not intended to be prescriptive, and is not only confined to an examination of practice, but can be seen as a means of making sense of experience by drawing on a range of documentary resources, asking questions and openly exploring theoretical ideas and possibilities with others. In thinking about debriefs, supervisions and tutorials it is important, as a learner, to be proactive, taking ideas, observations and questions to mentors, supervisors and tutors and not necessarily waiting for them to lead and guide. By adopting a curiously questioning and enquiring stance, we can develop as reflective learners and practitioners.

At a very basic level the key reflective questions are 'How?' and 'Why?'. Beckett and Hager (2002: 36) argue that the relationship between 'know how' and 'know why' is constantly under renegotiation through reflexive and reflective processes. Citing the work of Argyris and Schön they describe reflexivity as a process that 'encourages action, not merely reaction' and reflectivity as a process that 'encourages an interrogative stance to received views' (2002: 20). This means that as reflexive practitioners we adopt a position that commits us to taking action to improve our own performance, or the performance of the collective. This is important as sometimes reflexivity can appear to be a merely intellectual exercise. Reflectivity requires that we recognize that we do not operate in isolation, as individuals, work teams or university peer groups – we learn and practise within a social, cultural and political context. These interlocking contexts generate local, regional and national policy and practice. Sometimes, in reflective mode, we have to question policies and practices. Such questions may be to develop our understanding; sometimes they may be to challenge 'how things are'. The purpose however is always directed towards some sort of improvement in the conditions of those with whom we work, or within ourselves.

Various authors have proposed a range of reflective questions and processes that practitioners can use to guide themselves and/or others. Winter and Munn-Giddings (2001) synthesize an array of questions drawn from the writings of a number of educationists. They take us from the basics of 'What happened, what surprised me and why?' through to a form of dialectics. Fish *et al.* (1991) take the learner and facilitator through a very systematic and thorough process of 'sorting out the facts', or 'telling the story'. This involves critically analysing the story told – examining it for patterns, thinking about how others might have perceived the event and hypothesizing relevant knowledge.

Throughout the literature, questions posed by authors have a significant degree of similarity, with some adding particular perspectives, dependent on their specialist concerns or interests. Johns (1999), for example, introduces us to an ethical and aesthetic perspective. Any or all of the questions can be helpful, none carry greater weight than any others and practitioners may find it beneficial to 'play around' within them. The most useful aspect of all the available models is the structure they lend to the examination of learning and experience. These frameworks for guided reflection can help us analyse experience on a regular basis, without being dependent on the inspirational flash of insight. Nonetheless, those inspirational revelations that come to mind on waking or while making supper can be of equal value and significance and should not be dismissed – it is always useful to jot them down if they are not to be acted upon immediately.

There is no one way to develop as a reflective practitioner or to develop a reflective practice. A variety of paths or techniques are available to us. We can keep a reflective journal and on many professional courses this is a requirement (Thorpe 2004). We can explore our experience and thinking through formal one-to-one supervisory sessions. We can engage in the reflective process as a member of a group.

Group reflections do not necessarily require everyone to examine the same issues. Individuals can bring their own concerns to a group as long as there is a willingness to ask appropriate reflective questions, listen to the individual and help them pursue their thinking as far as possible (Winter *et al*. 1999).

A reflective stance locates us within a feedback loop, albeit either personal to ourselves or public as part of a learning and teaching strategy. Effective reflective practitioners need to listen, observe and make notes of the things that catch their attention so that they can return to them for greater scrutiny later, consider the perspectives of others and ask curious questions about how things are known and how things are. Having collected our data we need to determine our next step forward and commence the reflective cycle again. Very often our reflective processes are not explicit to us but are part of the 'hot action' (Beckett and Hager 2002: 23) of the practice experience as it unfolds. As Beckett and Hager argue, it is also useful to look back in order to move forward, asking 'what are we doing, why are we doing it, what comes next?'

Presenting your learning

At various points in the course of our studies – and work lives – we are required to provide accounts of our learning to our teachers and our peers. Presenting our learning, knowledge and ideas – either orally or in written form – is an aspect of genuinely reflective practice; it engages us in sharing and learning with others. As has been discussed, much of our learning is demonstrated implicitly in seminars, tutorials, supervisions and in direct practice with service users. Sometimes, however, we need to evidence what we have learned through formal media such as written assignments and presentations. Whichever format we are required to produce there are two key features that must be taken into account: audience and structure.

Audience

In communicating with an audience the greatest need is for clarity, of both purpose and expression. The audience needs to be convinced that the content of a presentation is relevant and worthwhile, and they need to be able to understand what is being said. So, the structure of a presentation has to be logical (with a beginning, middle and end), and the language used should be clear, precise and jargon-free. Where there is a need for technical or professional language it is sensible to explain basic concepts in simple terms. In both written and oral presentations, setting out definitions is a useful thing to do as these provide a solid foundation or framework for the rest of the material. Equally, it is also important to ensure that the work we present is error free – for example, spelling and grammar should be correct; factual content should be accurate; all sources of material should be assiduously attributed. Errors have the potential to undermine the confidence of the audience, and so are to be avoided at all costs.

When speaking to a live audience we need to be sure that we can be heard by everyone in the room – speaking clearly and with authority is critical to 'holding' an audience. On some occasions particular technologies may be required for those who are hearing impaired or deaf, or those with visual impairments. As well as by speaking clearly, confidence can be demonstrated by ensuring that everyone can see you (so maybe stand up rather than sit) and by adopting open and receptive body language. This means making eye contact with individuals in the room, listening attentively when asked questions and responding thoughtfully rather than defensively to audience comments. In situations where the audience is encouraged to participate – which can be useful for judging how ideas are understood and received by others – it is not necessary to always have an answer or response. The audience may contribute ideas or raise questions that you had not considered and it is acceptable to acknowledge this and even thank individuals for their contribution to your own thinking.

Structure

The fundamental formula for structuring presentations was set down by the classical rhetorician Quintilian (1921). The principles he set out still apply in the modern world and can be summed up as:

- a brief introduction;
- a statement that lays out the key content or focus of the presentation (Quintilian described these as 'narrative' or 'propositional' statements);
- the core of the presentation where the arguments or reasons in support of the description or analysis offered are discussed;
- a conclusion that sums up all that has already been said.

With live audiences, skilled presenters often begin with a light-hearted comment or banter in introducing themselves and the topic, with the remaining aspects of a presentation sometimes summarized as, 'Tell them what you are going to tell them; then tell them what you are telling them; then tell them what you told them.' This works because it has a clear explanatory basis through which complex information can be delivered. Audiences, particularly when listening to oral presentations, cannot remember the information being conveyed unless it is repeated. These structural principles also apply when writing texts.

Reflection point

Think about how you can prepare for your next oral presentation, taking into account the following.

- The length of time you have available to communicate your key information or message.
- The knowledge and experience of your audience.
- The ways in which you can enhance your personal confidence in undertaking the presentation (e.g. being sure of the facts; being up to date with reading and literature; rehearsing the presentation).

Conclusion

Whether in the classroom or in the practice setting, learning and teaching take place in a complex context and as learners we are exposed to a range of external and internal stimuli. In order to make sense of this raw data and learn from it we need to:

- recognize that learning and teaching is an ongoing interaction between learners, teachers and service users that requires us to open ourselves up to dialogue with others;
- acknowledge the complexity of the learning environment and aim to forge constructive relationships with others who may think differently to ourselves;
- adopt an holistic and authentic approach to communicating with others so that we can listen to, and be open to, the exploration of new, or even 'tried and tested' ideas;
- take advantage of learning opportunities wherever they arise and respectfully seek them out through purposeful negotiations with teaching teams and service users;
- develop our capacity as reflective learners and practitioners, seeking to improve or change our personal performance, or that of the collective.

References

Ashcroft, K. and Foreman-Peck, L. (1994) *Managing Teaching and Learning in Further and Higher Education*. London: Falmer Press.

Barrington, K. and Street, K. (2008) Learner contracts in nurse education: interaction within the practice context, *Nurse Education in Practice*, 9: 109–18.

Beckett, D. and Hager, P. (2002) *Life, Work and Learning: Practice in Postmodernity*. London: Routledge.

Cottrell, S. (2005) *Critical Thinking Skills*. Basingstoke: Palgrave Macmillan.

Edgecombe, K. and Bowden, M. (2009) The ongoing search for best practice in clinical teaching and learning: a model of nursing students' evolution to proficient novice registered nurses, *Nurse Education in Practice*, 9: 91–101.

Ekeburgh, M. (2009) Developing a didactic method that emphasises lifeworld as a basis for learning, *Reflective Practice*, 10(1): 51–63.

Fanthorne, C. (2004) *Work Placements: A Survival Guide for Students*. Basingstoke: Palgrave Macmillan.

Fish, D., Twinn, S. and Purr, B. (1991) *Promoting Reflection: Improving the Supervision of Practice in Health Visiting and Initial Teacher Training*. London: West London Institute.

Freire, P. (1972) *Pedagogy of the Oppressed*. Harmondsworth: Penguin.

Hanley, P. (2009) Communication skills in social work, in R. Adams, L. Dominelli and M. Payne (eds) *Social Work: Themes, Issues and Critical Debates*, 3rd edn. Basingstoke: Palgrave Macmillan.

Johns, C. (1999) Unravelling the dilemmas within everyday nursing practice, *Nursing Ethics*, 6(4): 287–98.

Knewstubb, B. and Bond, C. (2009) What's he talking about? The communicative alignment between a teacher's understanding and students' understanding, *Higher Education Research and Development*, 28(2): 179–93.

Kolb, D.A. (1984) *Experiential Learning: Experience as the Source of Learning and Development.* Englewood Cliffs, NJ: Prentice Hall.

Laitinen-Vaananen, S., Talvitie, P. and Minna-Riitta, L. (2007) Clinical supervision as an interaction between the clinical educator and the student, *Physiotherapy and Practice,* 23(2): 95–103.

McCabe, C. (2004) Nurse-patient communication: an exploration of patients' experiences, *Journal of Clinical Nursing,* 13: 41–9.

McCroskey, L.L., Richmond, V.P. and McCroskey, J.C. (2002) The scholarship of teaching and learning: contributions from the discipline of communication, *Communication Education,* 51(4): 383–91.

Mezirow, J. (1991) *Transformative Dimensions of Adult Learning.* San Francisco: Jossey-Bass.

NMC (Nursing and Midwifery Council) (2008) *The Code: Standards of Conduct, Performance and Ethics for Nurses and Midwives,* www.nmc-uk.org.uk (accessed 11 March 2010).

Payne, C.J. and Scott, T. (1982) *Developing Supervision of Teams in Field and Residential Work: Part I.* London: National Institute of Social Work.

Quintilian, M.F. (1921) *Instituto Oratoria,* trans. H.E. Butler, Book IV. London: Loeb Classical Library.

Smith, M.K. (2004) Carl Rogers and informal education, in *The Encyclopaedia of Informal Education,* www.infed.org/thinkers/et-rogers.htm (accessed 25 June 2009).

Thorpe, K. (2004) Reflective learning journals: from concept to practice, *Reflective Practice,* 5(3): 327–43.

WIAL (World Institute for Action Learning) (2009) www.wial.org (accessed 19 July 2009).

Winter, R. and Munn-Giddings, C. (2001) *Handbook for Action Research in Health and Social Care.* London: Routledge.

Winter, R., Buck, A. and Sobiechowska, P. (1999) *Professional Experience and the Investigative Imagination: The Art of Reflective Writing.* London: Routledge.

9 | Legal and ethical dimensions in communication

Bernard Anderson

When communicating with patients, families, carers and colleagues, it is essential we consider our practice from both legal and ethical perspectives. This chapter will consider the nature of ethics and how this is related to nursing practice. We will then proceed to consider ethics and communication more generally. Specific issues such as consent, record-keeping and confidentiality are raised in the context of daily nursing practice, actively encouraging nurses to consider the ethical dilemmas that can result from our everyday encounters.

Learning outcomes

By the end of this chapter you should be able to:
1 Develop an understanding of the ethical dimensions of communication.
2 Become aware of the problems associated with providing truthful and accurate information for patients concerning their conditions and management.
3 Recognize the importance of confidentiality when dealing with sensitive patient information.

What is ethics?

Pose the question, 'What is ethics?' in the context of healthcare and often the answer given will relate to serious matters linked with euthanasia or other issues concerning end of life decisions, the treatment of very premature babies or the allocation of scarce resources or expensive treatments. These issues make the practical nature of ethics clear – however, although we may encounter such examples in the media they are often remote from our everyday experience.

We can look at more fundamental and yet simpler answers to this question. Ethics is concerned with two important and related ideas – providing benefit and avoiding harm, the principles of beneficence and non-maleficence. These are two of the principles mentioned by Beauchamp and Childress (2009) in the most recent edition of what has become one of the most widely used and cited books on the subject of biomedical ethics, but they are also mentioned more specifically in the context of interpersonal communication by Englehardt (2001).

As the latter author notes, these two principles indicate that it is possible to assess the quality of any decision or action in terms of the benefit or harm that results from it. Actions are judged to be good in as much as they promote benefit or avoid harm and bad in as much as they do not. Since these principles can be widely applied, it is clear that ethics is not confined to such complex questions as mentioned above but is far more extensive. In his introductory book on moral philosophy, Billington (1993) suggests any action which affects the welfare of another, however remotely, has an ethical dimension and hence requires assessment from an ethical perspective.

This identifies a further thread in ethics, namely a concern with the justification or rationale given for actions affecting others. Such justification, whether made on an individual basis by the person concerned when making a choice between two or more possibilities, or by those who require an explanation for the choice made, is typically made in terms of the benefits that result or the harms that are avoided.

Another way of thinking about ethics is to consider it in terms of guidance and advice. Again this frequently uses the application of these two principles. This is the approach underlying the codes of conduct that have been developed by professional organizations including the Nursing and Midwifery Council (NMC) (2008). These and other pieces of supplementary advice indicate both the priorities that should guide choices in action and also what should be appropriate action for a professional who is charged with protecting the welfare of others.

As already noted, one author, Englehardt (2001), has written about the importance of the ethical dimension of interpersonal communication. Her book considers this aspect of communication in normal human interactions. Healthcare in general and nursing care in particular depend on effective communication and as a result the way in which nurses communicate with others, including their patients, influences their patients' welfare.

It is important to recognize that there is an inevitability and uncertainty about communication. It does not only occur when and in the way in which we intend but can be entirely unintentional. The ethical dimensions of intentional communication are easy to appreciate: if we take time to deal with others in a sensitive and considerate fashion, then the aim to promote their welfare and avoid causing harm, for example by offence or insult, is clear. Similarly, if we are curt and dismissive our disregard for the feelings of the other person is also clear. However, there are other areas of interaction where the intention is less clear. Unintentional communication covers such areas as misunderstandings and misinterpretation but also unconscious actions such as fidgeting or looking at a watch, and those areas over which we have less control such as some facial expressions. All of these convey information to the recipient. Awareness of the possibility of unintentional communication is as important as consideration of the impact of intentional communication.

Ethical issues in non-verbal communication

How can unintentional communication affect the welfare of others? Consider the following example.

Vignette   Keeping up appearances

Aisha is in the second year of her nurse training. She moved to live in university accommodation from where she travels to her placements. It is the first time that she has lived away from home and has had to take responsibility for her day-to-day living arrangements. She is considered to be a competent and caring nurse. When she is getting ready to travel to the hospital for her shift one morning she realizes that her uniform dress is rather crumpled, but as she has to catch a bus she does not have time to iron it. She arrives at work on time but her unironed dress makes her look rather unkempt.

Is the state of Aisha's dress an ethical issue? On one level no – she is on time and ready for work, and she is likely to be able to complete her work in a satisfactory manner despite looking rather untidy. She is judged a competent and caring nurse, which ought to be enough. She will gain experience in the delivery of care and also provide, as a part of this, some contribution to the care of patients. However, it is not merely a matter of being able to complete her work in a purely practical way. One aspect of her role is gaining and maintaining the trust of her patients – she is a representative of the nursing profession while at work. On this basis she runs the risk of creating a bad impression and undermining the confidence that patients and colleagues have in her. If patients are put off by her appearance, or feel that she is behaving in an unprofessional way, she may not be able to gain their confidence and work as effectively. While this may seem trivial, consider the following patient perspective.

Patient perspective

The comments made by Lord Mancroft on his experience while a patient in hospital suggest that this unintentional aspect of non-verbal communication is more important than we might realize. Speaking in the House of Lords about his time in hospital he described nurses as 'mostly grubby, with dirty fingernails and hair . . . slipshod, lazy and worst of all drunken and promiscuous' (*Hansard* 2008). He went on to add that as a patient in hospital he noticed that when lying in bed with nurses on each side he felt that they spoke to each other as though he were not there.

Whether Lord Mancroft's observations are an accurate reflection of nurses and contemporary nursing practice can be debated; however, they are based on a patient's personal observations of nurses in practice, their appearance and conversations. They demonstrate the way behaviour and conversations are interpreted and understood by those around us and hence the importance of non-verbal communication. They also show that the most significant component of this can be entirely unintentional. Aisha, like many other nurses, would be mortified by an assessment such as Lord Mancroft's, however, it makes clear just how important attention to minor details can be.

Reflection point
- Was Aisha's approach and attitude unprofessional?
- Should her mentor comment on the importance of being smartly turned out?

Even if we think of ourselves as open minded and liberal in our attitudes, we still have clear expectations of those who present themselves to us as professionals. We expect them to be courteous and neatly dressed, to notice that we are present and conduct themselves in what we consider to be an appropriate fashion. This is often conditioned and conventional but that does not make it unimportant. While we may be happy to talk to a car mechanic in oily overalls or discuss our plans for home improvements with a builder in clothes which indicate he has just come from another job, we would not be comfortable to see a consultant surgeon or a nurse in a clinic wearing blood-spattered clothing. As noted above, this is not just a nicety but a reflection of what we consider to be reasonable expectations and a means of gaining our trust. In addition to being competent in a practical sense, Aisha needs to recognize and meet the expectations of her patients in terms of her appearance.

A further aspect of interactions with patients at this level concerns the way we react to them and their problems. Most of us feel either frightened or awkward when we need to seek the support and help of others in relation to our health. We feel reassured by professionals who are not disturbed by our medical problems but take them in their stride.

Vignette   Establishing trust and confidence

Carly was asked to attend to Simeon, who was recovering from major surgery for bowel cancer. He had a colostomy and a wound infection. Simeon was not yet able to attend to his own colostomy and both this and the wound infection gave rise to very unpleasant odours. Grace was asked to assist Carly and when the dressing was to be removed for changing, Grace immediately looked away, murmured that she could not stay and promptly left the room.

As with Aisha in the first vignette, there is an ethical dimension involved here. A key element of providing nursing care is that of being able to establish and maintain the trust and confidence of patients. Simeon needs to feel his problems are not so awful that others cannot cope, especially those who are expected to deal with his care. A nurse who induces concern or embarrassment in her patients by her reactions is behaving in a way that is in a very real sense unethical, in much the same way as the flight attendant who lost her nerve in unexpected turbulence on a transatlantic flight and began screaming, 'We're crashing!'. One of the passengers commented later that passengers expect flight attendants to be able to reassure them in such situations rather than induce uncertainty and panic (Hickman 2006).

Both Aisha's crumpled dress and Grace's sudden departure reflect unintentional rather than intentional communication and should be judged accordingly. In another context they would simply be regarded as aspects of professional etiquette, rather than being seen as communication. It should be clear that this distinction is more imaginary than real and that lack of attention to detail or sudden and unexpected reactions by nurses and other health professionals can be interpreted as disinterest or distaste by those who depend on them. Medicine has been described as a paradoxical art (Weston 2009) and nursing can be viewed in the same way. Gabriel Weston suggests that a good doctor needs to be able to get close enough to patients for them to feel able to disclose important and personal information and yet remain distant enough to be unaffected. Nursing is similarly paradoxical.

Ethical issues in verbal communication

The use of language in verbal communication makes the whole process seem simpler and more straightforward. Verbal communication is more obviously concerned with gathering and providing information and as a result we can think of it as being intentional rather than unintentional. However, as with non-verbal communication, mutual trust and respect are central. There are two key areas:

- truthfulness in disclosure;
- consent before intervention.

Both of these can be linked with another of the principles outlined by Beauchamp and Childress – respect for autonomy. Truthfulness involves honesty and requires that patients are given information that is comprehensive, accurate and objective. As in the case of the general question at the beginning about the nature of ethics, information disclosure most frequently prompts us to think about the disclosure of bad news in relation to diagnosis and prognosis. However, it can arise in other instances as well.

> **Vignette   Medication error**
>
> Manshi and Samantha were preparing to give Joyce an intravenous injection of an antibiotic. This was the last of several injections to be given. As her blood results indicated renal failure, the dose of the antibiotic had been reduced. Neither Manshi nor Samantha noticed this while they were preparing the drug and as a result Joyce was given the full dose. Once they realized their error they recorded it and reported it to both the medical staff and the pharmacy. Coincidentally, Joyce's renal function returned to normal. Manshi was advised that in view of this, and in the light of the fact that it was the last dose, no further action was needed.

Aside from any questions about how attentive Manshi and Samantha were to correct procedures, it is relevant to ask whether Joyce should have been told that she had received the wrong dose of the right drug. We can surmise that she will not suffer any ill effects. If she does not ask, do we need to tell her? One approach to the question is to say that in the interests of honesty and openness the information should be volunteered. The justification for this could be made on the basis that it is important to keep patients informed in order to maintain their trust. If patients are not kept informed and told the truth about what is happening to them they are unlikely to trust those who care for them.

Alternatively, we can argue that this approach, though open, seems brutally honest and it is legitimate to ask whether Joyce gains anything as a result of the disclosure. It could do more harm than good, as one of the effects may be to prompt her to wonder what else might have gone wrong or to feel that she cannot trust at least two members of the staff who have to care for her. What about the arguments for not telling her? We have already noted that the error will almost certainly not give rise to any harm. On that basis we can argue that disclosing the fact of the error provides little benefit to Joyce, and furthermore in not knowing the truth she will not suffer any harm.

Reflection point
- If you were Joyce, how would you feel if you had been told of the error?
- How would you feel if you were not told but discovered it by accident later?
- If you were Manshi or Samantha, how would you have handled this situation?

More issues in disclosure

Disclosure of clinical information related to diagnosis and prognosis has traditionally been seen as the responsibility of medical rather than nursing staff. However, nursing staff may well be caught up in these processes and not infrequently asked questions that come to patients at times when medical colleagues are not available.

Vignette   Honesty and truthfulness

Gemma is 35 and has two young children. She has been admitted to the ward for treatment of a severe chest infection. In the course of routine checks on her progress it is discovered that the infection has been masking what appears to be a tumour. Gemma is now to undergo further investigation to determine whether this is the case and what other treatment is appropriate. Before the medical staff come to see her she asks one of the nurses how she is progressing and when she is likely to be discharged.

Activity

Consider the following in relation to the previous vignette.

- How would you respond to Gemma?
- What might be the impact of telling her that you weren't sure but that the doctor would come to see her as soon as possible?

Gemma is unaware of the underlying problem. The issue for us to consider is what she should be told and, further, what amounts to an honest and truthful answer. In the light of what the staff know, it is possible to treat an answer such as 'I am not sure, we need to check with the doctor' as truthful, but given what we suspect, is it really open and honest? If she is subsequently told that she needs to be investigated further because of the suspicion of a tumour, she may surmise (accurately) that the nursing staff have not been entirely honest with her. As a result, her confidence in them would be undermined. Alternatively, if she is told that she needs to undergo further investigation, the nurses may not be clear what this entails or when it will take place, and consequently Gemma would be left confused and worried. Telling the truth, superficially a simple matter, turns out to be much more complex than we might imagine.

In many situations like this, there are two separate questions:

- What amounts to a truthful answer?
- How much information should patients be given?

The first question raises important philosophical issues which lie outside the scope of this chapter. However, a flavour of this can be gained by considering a case reported in the medical journal *The Lancet*. In a letter to the journal a doctor described an encounter with a man who had a cancerous but easily cured ulcer on his lip (Brewin 1994). The patient, who was clearly frightened, asked whether he had cancer. His doctor realized that although the patient did have cancer, he did not have what the patient *understood* by cancer and gave a negative answer to the man's question. Although this was untrue it was actually an honest answer to the question posed. Although it is tempting to think of truth as certain it is often less precise and clear than we imagine. This example also illustrates the importance of being aware of the meaning of the question rather than simply the literal meaning of the words. The way in which the question is interpreted and understood by the listener is important and careful attention to the real meaning rather than simply the obvious one is vital, not merely from a practical perspective but also from an ethical one.

A further complication arises in relation to the differing interpretations attached to ideas such as honesty, frankness and directness, by both patients and professionals and also by different individuals. In an interesting and sometimes rather provocative book based on his experiences as a consultant working in a large city hospital Tallis (2004) observes that one person's honesty is another's brutal frankness and what for one is direct communication is perceived as crass indifference to the feelings and wellbeing of another by someone else. Ethical communication can be, and often is, fraught with difficulty.

The scope of disclosure, or more simply, the amount of information provided to patients, is also a difficult issue. It can be managed by what is termed 'staged' or 'incremental' disclosure. Information is provided in small amounts in response to questions asked by the patient rather than all of it being given at one time. As a means of communication this is useful as it allows the patient to set the pace and enables disclosure and the provision of information to take the form of a dialogue rather than being an event.

Patient perspective

In writing of his own experience the late John Diamond, who was both a columnist on a national newspaper and a television journalist, makes it beautifully clear that, from a patient perspective, incremental disclosure may be less than satisfactory. Information may need to be drawn from the professional or worse be discovered by chance rather than as a result of a planned open dialogue (Diamond 1998). Reading his account there is no sense that any of the professionals were incompetent or unkind; rather that they failed to appreciate his need to be a partner and participant in the process of his own treatment and not merely a passive recipient of their expertise.

Consent

Consent is an aspect of care that is almost taken for granted by practitioners. Again, it is one in which communication is central. Consent is similar to giving permission. In the context of healthcare this may be for an examination or for some form of treatment or care. Seeking consent can operate on several levels. On one level we can think of it as a matter of common courtesy or good manners – we ask or warn before we act. From an ethical perspective, seeking consent before a procedure is a practical demonstration of respect for others and a recognition that their goals, preferences and choices may differ from those of the professional who is offering a service. This again reflects the principle of respect for a patient's autonomy.

From a legal perspective, consent is important because touching another person without permission is a form of trespass and, therefore, unlawful. Consequently, for medical and nursing procedures to be lawful, consent is important as it is the normal defence for trespass. Since some care and treatment can take place over extended periods of time it is useful to think of consent in terms of enduring permission, or taking the form of a dialogue in which the patient's willingness to proceed is checked at intervals. Although this is most obviously the case in extended treatments, it is worth using this definition of consent as enduring permission more generally, as it takes into account the fact that patients may have a change of mind at any time before a procedure actually takes place. It is also important to recognize that consent is quite different from acquiescence; it cannot be concluded that consent has been given simply because a patient did not obviously object to what was being done.

We often think of consent in terms of the written consent obtained by the completion of the commonly used consent forms, but this is best seen as an end point of a process, which includes providing information, discussion and decision-making (DH 2001). Indeed, written consent is not the only form of consent, so a consent form is best seen as a record of consent having been given at a particular time. Viewing consent as a process rather than an event makes it clear that communication has a fundamental role to play.

Obtaining valid consent involves three key elements:

- assessment of capacity;
- disclosure of information;
- checking that consent is being freely given.

Communication is important in each of these but most significant in the second – disclosure of information. Communication is relevant from two different but related perspectives:

- the amount of information provided;
- the level of understanding.

How much information should be provided for a patient? The aim of disclosure is to help the patient to make a decision rather than simply provide information to satisfy curiosity or fill a gap in a patient's knowledge. In simple terms, to give valid consent, patients need to know the nature, purpose and likely effects of any proposed action or treatment. Put another way, patients need to know what is going to be done or given, why and what they might expect to happen as a result. It is also important to tell patients what might happen if the proposed course of action is not followed and whether there are viable alternatives to the treatment proposed.

Presented in this way, providing information for patients appears deceptively easy.

Patient perspective

Tallis (2004) mentions an article in a national newspaper in which Liz Kendall described her reactions to the 'routine' transfer of information described above. She records her relief that having described her symptoms, the consultant surgeon took her seriously, but laments his poor communication skills – highlighted by an ill-judged attempt to make witty remarks (unintentional communication). She goes on to list a host of unasked and hence unanswered questions she had after the consultation and wonders whether the consultant ought not to have been aware of these possible questions and hence have anticipated the need for this information (Kendall 2002).

Aside from the problem of accurately anticipating the questions a patient might need or wish to ask, Tallis points out that attempting to answer even some of these questions would be both time consuming and could be counter-productive. Rather than assisting the patient to make the decision, the patient might become confused and find the decision more difficult. Withholding information in a way that misleads a patient is clearly unethical, however, a compromise may be necessary since maximal disclosure may not serve the primary aim of helping patients make decisions they feel are appropriate. Striking this balance involves careful assessment and ethical judgement.

What then of the level of understanding? Knowledge without understanding is of limited value and if patients have the former without acquiring the latter they are not in a position to give valid consent. It is important to be aware that patients may be given information which is difficult to understand; good examples of this are the risks associated with a particular procedure or the chances of its success. Risk is normally calculated from large groups and indicates the proportion of all those who undergo the treatment who can expect a particular outcome. However, in the context of seeking consent such figures have to be applied to individual cases. John Diamond, whose book has already been mentioned, comments on this and the difficulty and confusion that it creates, and goes on to observe that for an individual the chance of success and survival is 50:50 – treatment either works or it does not. Again the way in which such complex information is presented and explained to patients is more than just a matter of providing facts.

There is a further difficulty facing patients. Information may be provided in circumstances where they are at a disadvantage. For example, they may have to make a decision soon after being given news of an unexpected or suspected but feared diagnosis. In such situations, nurses have an important role in assisting communication since they have a better understanding of the information given to patients and more opportunity to discuss things with them or seek clarification on their behalf when misunderstanding arises. The nurse thus takes on the responsibilities both of a chaperone and an advocate. These roles, however, are not without their own problems.

Patient perspective

The late Gillian Rose, who like John Diamond ultimately died from cancer, was determined that she be told the results of her surgery and also that she be involved in the decisions associated with her treatment. At one point she writes of the 'carnival of communication' that arose as a result of differences of interpretation of the same information among professionals and hence the most appropriate course of action (Rose 1995).

In this instance nurses were not involved but the point is an important one since what Rose comments on is the failure of the different professionals to understand each other and ultimately the needs and best interests of their patient.

Gabriel Weston, a surgeon, provides a further interesting insight into the way in which patient and professional expectations may differ. She describes an occasion when she needed to obtain consent from a young woman who was to have a bilateral mastectomy. Weston suggested that a less invasive procedure was possible and then ventured to suggest that reconstructive surgery could be considered. The patient did not wish to explore either of these, preferring instead to proceed with the radical surgery, but did wish to preserve the small mole that lay between her breasts (Weston 2009).

Although in general it is seen as the responsibility of medical staff to seek the consent of patients for the more important procedures, particularly if explicit and written consent is required, it may fall to the nurse to ensure that consent has been given and to check that the patient has not had second thoughts or is labouring under a misapprehension or misunderstanding.

Vignette   Valid consent (1)

James was admitted following investigations for suspected bowel cancer. He gave consent for surgery when he was reviewed prior to admission. However, it becomes clear as you talk to him when making final preparations for him to go to surgery that he is not fully aware of the possibility that he could have a permanent colostomy formed during surgery.

Activity

In relation to James's case:

- Can the nurse assume that James has given consent?
- If she has doubts what should she say to her colleagues in the operating theatre who may be expecting the arrival of James in the near future?

Although James has completed the necessary paperwork and is in hospital, has he actually given his consent? If nothing is said and the surgery goes ahead it could prove difficult for James to demonstrate from a legal perspective that he was not in agreement with the procedure. However, in a situation such as this it is difficult, despite the completion of the relevant consent form, to argue that James has given valid consent. If the surgery does go ahead it will be legal but unethical.

Consent covers more than simply gaining permission to carry out a specific procedure, typically a surgical intervention. It also involves willingness on the patient's part to cooperate in what is proposed and in this context the level of disclosure and the way information is provided may differ.

Vignette   Valid consent (2)

Alma has been referred by her GP with what appears to be chronic venous ulceration on her right leg. She has not previously been seen by any of the health service staff in the area. Following an assessment it is concluded that the most effective way of managing her ulcer is to apply compression bandages, as these will improve the venous return and offer the best chance of long-term healing.

Communication Skills for Adult Nurses

Activity

Think about Alma's case.

- Is her consent necessary?
- If it is, what information should she be given?

In this case we could just follow the model used above and outline the proposed treatment, its justification and the anticipated outcome. Would that be enough? On a superficial level the answer would be yes, however, for the treatment to succeed we need to enlist the cooperation of the patient. So additional information is required. Specifically Alma needs to know what is expected of her in order for the proposed treatment to be successful. As compression bandaging may be constricting and is often bulky, she will need to know both that it may be uncomfortable and may make it impossible for her to wear ordinary shoes. The technical superiority of the treatment takes on a different appearance when the full impact is outlined. In this and many other situations which involve longer-term interventions, the impact of the intervention on everyday life needs to be understood and communication requires a meeting of minds rather than just the exchange of ideas, since the latter can all too easily result in patients and professionals talking at, or even past, each other, rather than sharing information.

Written communication

Visit any doctor's surgery, any hospital clinic or ward and records of some sort will be visible. Traditionally records were kept on sheets of paper or pieces of card, but increasingly these have been replaced by some form of electronic storage but can still be considered written records and communication.

Why is record-keeping and written communication important? There are two reasons:

- It is a means of inter- and intraprofessional communication.
- It allows a historical account of what care has been given and the reasons for it.

The different professionals involved in delivering care need to communicate with each other on a day-to-day basis. As a result it should come as no surprise that the NMC makes this point in its guidance on record-keeping (NMC 2009). Such communication may be direct, if for example the written record is the only source of information available, or indirect and supplementary if the written record serves as a prompt for the professional when passing on information to another, or when the information is a useful addition to information provided in some other way. The value of this supplementary form of information was noted by the National Patient Safety Agency (NPSA) (2007a), when it reported that staff do not always adequately inform each other concerning patient care at times such as handover and transfer.

The value of a historical account is that it can assist either in recall should this be necessary, or in making further decisions at a later stage. For these reasons record-keeping is important. Furthermore, rather than simply being a practical activity which is all too often seen as a ritual or a chore, record-keeping, like other aspects of communication, has an important ethical dimension.

What are the problems with written communication and the ethical issues that arise?

- Records may be incomplete.
- The significance of the information may not be understood.

The value of complete records seems self-evident. If written information is a principal or the only source of information it is important that it is as comprehensive as possible. If not then decisions based on those records could be affected and the patient's care compromised as a result. Hence, accurate written accounts following assessment or the delivery of nursing care are an integral part of practice, rather than an optional element which can be added if and when time or inclination permits (NMC 2009). The importance of this was again reported by the NPSA (NPSA 2007a) where it was noted that incomplete and inadequate documentation was a contributing factor in the failure to recognize or respond to the seriousness of a patient's condition.

Vignette   Record-keeping

Martin reports for duty after two days away from the ward. He is given a handover for a group of patients. Two patients have been admitted since he was last on duty. He records key details in a small notebook that he carries with him. When he checks the documentation for one of the patients, he sees that since the beginning of the last shift no recordings have been made for temperature, blood pressure and fluid output, and concludes that the patient no longer requires this level of observation. Subsequently, the patient's condition deteriorates rapidly and Martin then discovers that the patient should have been managed differently.

The above vignette indicates both the importance of written information and the confusion that can arise when it is incomplete. Obviously, Martin could have asked other staff who were more familiar with the patient to confirm what needed to be done if he was unsure. However, in his defence he might argue that the absence of recordings indicated that they were no longer required and that he should be able to depend on such supplementary information as an indication of the type of care that was required.

Activity

In the case of Martin and the incomplete records, consider the following.

- When two sets of information are incompatible, how should we decide which to trust?
- If you had been in Martin's position, would you have acted differently?

In Martin's case the absence of records gave a false impression and resulted in inappropriate care. This example shows the importance of written communication in the provision of what one might consider routine care. It is also important in the case of untoward occurrences.

Let us return to consider the incident mentioned in the vignette on page 147, in which a patient was accidentally given an incorrect dose of the correct drug. The temptation is to think of this as just an untoward incident − the patient was accidentally given an incorrect dose of the drug − and to think of the appropriate means of recording this as the completion of the relevant incident form. However, thinking of it in this way misses an important point. The occurrence is something that others involved with the care of the patient need to know. Therefore, what happened, who was notified and the actions taken in response to any advice given need to be carefully documented. Then if contrary to advice and expectations there is a delayed adverse response, there is a clear account of the dose of the drug the patient was given and what action was subsequently taken.

Lack of understanding of what has been recorded or why it needs to be recorded is also an issue. A characteristic of medicine and nursing, as indeed of many other areas of activity, is the technical language and nomenclature involved. It is tempting to imagine that life would be much simpler without it. Unfortunately, this is not the case. While for those who do not understand it technical language is confusing, it serves an important function as it enables effective communication between those who use it as a matter of routine. The same is true for standard abbreviations and acronyms. As with other forms of communication, record-keeping is most effective when conventions are understood and followed (see Chapter 3).

A further problem arises when those who gather the information are inexperienced or have little understanding of the purpose and importance of the information gathered. If accurate and complete information is not understood and its importance and significance not appreciated, the welfare of the patient is put at risk and, as noted earlier, this is an important ethical issue not merely a practical one. Again this was noted by the NPSA (2007b) which reported that important signs of deterioration had been missed despite accurate recording of appropriate information and as a result patients were put at serious risk. Record-keeping had become an end in itself rather than a means to some other end.

Confidentiality

Much of what has been said so far has stressed the importance of communication, understood as the exchange of information. Effective patient care demands the free exchange of information between patient and professionals, between different professionals and different groups of professionals. This free exchange of information is important for the welfare of the patient. However, information is often sensitive and in order to protect the interests of patients, both gathering and sharing such information needs to be carefully managed. While once this was taken for granted both gathering and sharing personal information are now regulated by law through the Data Protection Act (1998) and its associated guidelines.

Key issues in information-gathering include:

- protection of confidentiality;
- whether the information is essential;
- the accuracy of the information.

Often the first thing that comes to mind in the context of gathering and managing personal information is the idea of confidentiality. However, before we can consider confidentiality, we need to think about what information should be obtained from patients or, if necessary, from their friends and family members. As a general rule, only information that is needed in order to deliver effective care should be gathered and this broad principle is reflected in the Data Protection Act (1998) and the associated data protection principles, particularly the third one which states that personal data shall be adequate, relevant and not excessive given the purpose for which it is gathered (see Chapter 4). The fourth principle requires that such information shall be accurate and, where necessary, kept up to date. These principles allow considerable scope for information collection, since it is not always clear what information might be needed – for example, in relation to previous health problems or current living arrangements.

As mentioned above, confidentiality is an important aspect of the patient–professional relationship which for medicine is considered to date back to the time of Hippocrates (c. 450 BCE) and the clause in the Hippocratic oath which demands discretion in speech. In more recent times the code of practice issued by the NMC directs nurses in this issue. Applied in the strictest sense, confidentiality would mean that we could not share any information without the permission of the person from whom it is gathered. However, in the context of nursing practice, for most purposes we can rely on implied consent to share information with others involved in the care of the patient on a need-to-know basis. Importantly, this principle does not extend beyond that closed group, even to close family members. Where confidential information has to be made more widely available the relevant code of practice should be consulted or the advice of a Caldicott Guardian be sought.

Vignette   Friends, relatives and confidentiality

Jessica was admitted for minor surgery which necessitated a short stay in hospital. She gave her sister as next of kin. Before she is discharged there is a telephone call to the ward and the caller asks about her and says he is her boyfriend. The nurse who takes the call confirms that Jessica is on the ward and is expected to be discharged later the same day. When she relays the information to Jessica, she becomes angry and says that she broke off her relationship with him and is worried that he might now follow her home.

What seems like an answer to casual enquiry has in this case acquired a more menacing tone and suggests a breach of confidentiality. The previous vignette also makes it clear that even quite innocuous questions about patients need to be treated with caution. A young woman who visits a gynaecology clinic may not want her parents to collect her and someone who has had a blood test for HIV may be concerned about the information being disclosed even if the test was negative. Seemingly routine information is not always as innocent as it seems.

Conclusion

Communication involves the exchange of information but as we have seen this is often more complex than we might realize and we need to be alert to and aware of inadvertent messages as well as the obvious ones. We also need to recognize that communication is a skill which is never completely mastered. Always remember the following:

- The ethical dimension of communication should always be considered.
- The importance of unintentional non-verbal cues should never be underestimated when considering communication from an ethical perspective.
- Communication is a skill that must be developed and refined throughout a nurse's career.
- The concepts of honesty, truthfulness and disclosure may present the nurse with significant ethical dilemmas, and may lead to different interpretations of information.
- An understanding of the concepts of consent and confidentiality is essential.
- Record-keeping, in addition to its legal function, has an important ethical dimension.
- Legal and ethical dimensions of practice are supported by guidelines produced by organizations including the NMC and the Department of Health.

References

Beauchamp, T.L. and Childress, J.F. (2009) *Principles of Biomedical Ethics*, 6th edn. New York: Oxford University Press.

Billington, R. (1993) *Living Philosophy – An Introduction to Moral Thought*, 2nd edn. London: Routledge.

Brewin, T.B. (1994) Telling the truth, *The Lancet*, 343: 1512.

DH (Department of Health) (2001) *Good Practice in Consent Implementation Guide: Consent to Examination or Treatment*. London: DH.

Diamond, J. (1998) *C – Because Cowards Get Cancer Too*. London: Vermillion.

Englehardt, E. (2001) *Ethical Issues in Interpersonal Communication*. Fort Worth, TX: Harcourt College Publishers.

Hansard (2008) 28 February, column 825.

Hickman, M. (2006) Flight attendant panics as jet falls 8000 feet in seconds, *The Independent*, 28 February.

Kendall, E. (2002) How I fell foul of the NHS, *The Sunday Times*, 24 February.

NMC (Nursing and Midwifery Council) (2008) *The Code: Standards of Conduct, Performance and Ethics for Nurses and Midwives*, www.nmc-uk.org.uk (accessed 11 March 2010).

NMC (Nursing and Midwifery Council) (2009) *Record-keeping: Guidance for Nurses and Midwives*, www.nmc-uk.org.uk.

NPSA (National Patient Safety Agency) (2007a) *Recognising and Responding Appropriately to Early Signs of Deterioration in Hospitalised Patients*, www.npsa.nhs.uk (accessed 4 January 2010).

NPSA (National Patient Safety Agency) (2007b) *Safer Care for the Acutely Ill Patient: Learning from Serious Incidents*, www.npsa.nhs.uk (accessed 4 January 2010).

Rose, G. (1995) *Love's Work*. London: Chatto & Windus.

Tallis, R. (2004) *Hippocratic Oaths – Medicine and its Discontents*. London: Atlantic Books.

Weston, G. (2009) *Direct Red: A Surgeon's Story*. London: Jonathan Cape.

Afterword

This book has introduced the student nurse to the importance of effective communication in all aspects of their work. We hope that it has inspired you to observe your own practice and that of those around you, and to strive to create better relationships with patients and colleagues. We believe that to be effective, learning should be enjoyable and we hope that aspiration has also been met.

Communication skills are often regarded as innate, and it has often been assumed that nurses are naturally good communicators. However, it has been shown that there are special skills required in different aspects of a nurse's working life, and these will develop and be refined over the course of a nurse's career and in response to the changing demands of healthcare on the nurse's role. Moreover, we know these skills can be taught and learned, and are an established feature in modern healthcare education. It is also important that beyond registration, nurses accept the need to access continuing professional development (CPD) to keep these skills honed so that they do not unconsciously become complacent or less effective.

In this book we have touched on some of the areas where we think attention to communication skills is particularly needed, and which will enhance practice and improve the patient's experience most. Each chapter topic has had several books written about it, and thus for the student nurse we could only provide an introduction to the areas covered. It is our intention that the reflections and activities will have provided students with an enthusiasm for developing their communication skills further so that they can become true holistic practitioners.

When you next access healthcare as a service user, consider and notice how you feel, and how the actions of the staff make you feel. Do you enter the building with a spring in your step or are your hackles raised before you are even at the reception desk? Have previous encounters and experiences as a patient or service user influenced how you feel? Many high profile cases that hit the headlines are peppered with issues that relate back to poor communication – between individuals and between services. Many poor experiences and indeed tragedies might be avoided by strengthening communication between healthcare staff and their clients.

Further reading

Charlton, R. (ed.) (2007) *Learning to Consult.* Oxford: Radcliffe Publishing.

Ghaye, T. and Lillyman, S. (2000) *Reflection: Principles and Practice for Healthcare Professionals.* London: Quay Books.

Ghaye, T. and Lillyman, S. (2006) *Learning Journals and Critical Incidents*, 2nd edn. London: Quay Books.

Glasper, A., McEwing, G. and Richardson, J. (eds) (2009) *Foundation Skills for Caring.* Basingstoke: Palgrave Macmillan.

Kaufman, G. (2008) Patient assessment: effective consultation and history-taking, *Nursing Standard*, 23: 50.

Moulton, L. (2007) *The Naked Consultation.* Oxford: Radcliffe Publishing.

Stein-Parbury, J. (2009) *Patient and Person.* Chatswood, NSW: Elsevier.

Tan Jia Xing, J. (2009) The use of effective therapeutic skills in nursing practice, *Singapore Nursing Journal*, 36: 35–40.

Timmins, F. (2007) Communication skills, *Nurse Prescribing*, 5: 10.

Tuohy, D. (2003) Student nurse–older person communication, *Nurse Education Today*, 23: 19–26.

Useful resources

The Alzheimers Society Factsheets: http://alzheimers.org.uk/factsheets
BLISS, Blissymbol Communication UK, www.blissymbols.co.uk
British Sign Language (BSL), British Deaf Association, http://www.bda.org.uk
Makaton Vocabulary Development Project, www.makaton.org
Mayer Johnson Symbols, Mayer-Johnson LLC, www.mayer-johnson.com
Paget Gormon, Paget Gormon Society, www.pgss.org
Patient Voices, www.patientvoices.org.uk
Rebus, Widgit Software Ltd, www.widgit.com
Signalong, The Signalong Group, www.signalong.org.uk

Index

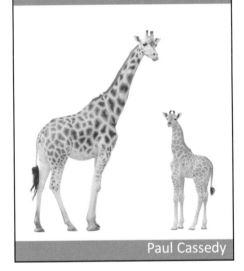

FIRST STEPS IN CLINICAL SUPERVISION

A Guide for Healthcare Professionals

Paul Cassedy

9780335236510 (Paperback)

November 2010

eBook also available

This practical book is designed as a toolkit for anyone starting out as a clinical supervisor. The book focuses on developing core skills of supervision, as well as your ability to reflect and improve on those skills.

Addressing all aspects of supervision, the book gives you practical frameworks needed to start, maintain and evaluate clinical supervision - from how to start a supervision contract to how to run a session.

Key features:

- Clear information and guidance on what the supervisor needs to know as they prepare to take on the role of clinical supervisor
- Practical examples and demonstration of key clinical supervision skills
- Simple explanations of the key frameworks and models for clinical supervision

www.openup.co.uk

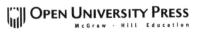

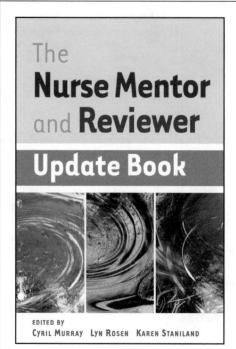

EDITED BY
CYRIL MURRAY LYN ROSEN KAREN STANILAND

THE NURSE MENTOR AND REVIEWER UPDATE BOOK

Cyril Murray, Lyn Rosen and
    Karen Staniland

9780335241194 (Paperback)
2010

eBook also available

This practical and flexible guide explains the meaning of competence and is designed to help mentors judge competence in line with Nursing and Midwifery Council standards and the NHS Knowledge and Skills Framework.

Key features:

- Designed to help mentors judge their own competence against national standards
- Supports qualified mentors in meeting the evidence required for annual updates
- A range of activities are included to help support the mentoring process to provide a range of different sources of evidence at appraisal interviews

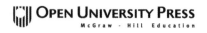 **OPEN UNIVERSITY PRESS**
McGraw - Hill Education

www.openup.co.uk